Promoting Self-Determination in Students with Developmental Disabilities

Developmental Disabilities

1593854609 -

Guilford Press c2007

WHAT WORKS FOR SPECIAL-NEEDS LEARNERS

Karen R. Harris and Steve Graham
Editors

Strategy Instruction for Students with Learning Disabilities
Robert Reid and Torri Ortiz Lienemann

Teaching Mathematics to Middle School Students
with Learning Difficulties
Marjorie Montague and Asha K. Jitendra, Editors

Teaching Word Recognition:
Effective Strategies for Students with Learning Difficulties
Rollanda E. O'Connor

Teaching Reading Comprehension to Students with Learning Difficulties
Janette K. Klingner, Sharon Vaughn, and Alison Boardman

Promoting Self-Determination
in Students with Developmental Disabilities
Michael L. Wehmeyer

Promoting Self-Determination in Students with Developmental Disabilities

Michael L. Wehmeyer

with

Martin Agran
Carolyn Hughes
James E. Martin
Dennis E. Mithaug
Susan B. Palmer

Series Editors' Note by Karen R. Harris and Steve Graham

THE GUILFORD PRESS
New York   London

©2007 The Guilford Press
A Division of Guilford Publications, Inc.
72 Spring Street, New York, NY 10012
www.guilford.com

Printed in the United States of America

This book is printed on acid-free paper.

Last digit is print number: 9   8   7   6   5   4   3   2   1

Library of Congress Cataloging-in-Publication Data

Wehmeyer, Michael L.
    Promoting self-determination in students with developmental disabilities / Michael L. Wehmeyer, with Martin Agran . . . [et al.].
        p. cm. — (What works for special-needs learners)
    Includes bibliographical references and index.
    ISBN-13: 978-1-59385-460-7 (pbk. : alk. paper)
    ISBN-10: 1-59385-460-9 (pbk. : alk. paper)
    ISBN-13: 978-1-59385-461-4 (hardcover : alk. paper)
    ISBN-10: 1-59385-461-7 (hardcover : alk. paper)
    1. Learning disabled children—Education.   2. Learning disabled youth—Education.   3. Decision making in children.   4. Decision making in adolescence.   5. Determination (Personality trait) in children.   I. Title.
    LC4704.W425 2007
    371.9—dc22
                                                            2007008172

About the Authors

Michael L. Wehmeyer, PhD, is Professor, Department of Special Education; Director, Kansas University Center on Developmental Disabilities; and Associate Director, Beach Center on Disability at the University of Kansas. He is the author of 195 refereed articles or book chapters and has authored or edited 20 books on disability- and education-related issues pertaining to self-determination, transition, universal design for learning and access to the general curriculum for students with severe disabilities, and technology use by people with cognitive disabilities. He is a member of the board of directors and a fellow of the American Association on Intellectual and Developmental Disabilities, a past president of the Council for Exceptional Children's (CEC) Division on Career Development and Transition, and editor-in-chief of *Remedial and Special Education*. In 1999 Dr. Wehmeyer was the inaugural recipient of the Distinguished Early Career Research Award from the CEC's Division for Research. In 2003 he received the National Education Award from the American Association on Intellectual and Developmental Disabilities. He holds undergraduate and master's degrees in special education from the University of Tulsa and a master's degree in experimental psychology from the University of Sussex in England, where he was a Rotary International Fellow. He earned his PhD in human development and communication sciences from the University of Texas at Dallas.

Martin Agran, PhD, is a Professor and Chair of the Department of Special Education at the University of Wyoming. Prior to this appointment, he was a department head at the University of Northern Iowa and a Professor in the Department of Special Education at Utah State University. Dr. Agran's areas of research are in self-determination and student-directed learning. He has published extensively in refereed journals and texts on these and other issues relating to the inclusion of students with severe disabilities, and has authored or coauthored 12 books. He is also an associate editor of *Research and Practice in Severe Disabilities* and is on the editorial board of *Education and Training in Developmental Disabilities*. Dr. Agran has served as a Fulbright Scholar in the Czech Republic and is currently serving as a consultant to Saratov University in Saratov, Russia. He was awarded the CEC's Division on Developmental Disabilities Research Award, the Donald McKay Research Award at the University of Northern Iowa, and the Thomas Haring Excellence in Research Award from TASH for outstanding research in the area of inclusive practice.

Carolyn Hughes, PhD, is Professor of Special Education and Human and Organizational Development, Peabody College of Education, at Vanderbilt University, and a research investigator in the John F. Kennedy Center at Vanderbilt. Dr. Hughes's research interests are in the transition to adult life for high-poverty youth, dropout prevention, self-determination and mentoring strategies for at-risk students and students with disabilities, and social interaction among general education high school students and their peers with disabilities. Dr. Hughes developed the Peabody Mentoring Program and has managed several federally funded projects, including the Metropolitan Nashville Peer Buddy Program, a service-learning program for general education students and their peers with disabilities. She is coauthor of *The Transition Handbook* and *Success for All Students: Promoting Inclusion in Secondary Schools through Peer Buddy Programs*. In addition, she has published numerous studies examining self-directed learning skills of high school students.

James E. Martin, PhD, holds the Zarrow Endowed Chair in Special Education and is Director of the Zarrow Center at the University of Oklahoma. Dr. Martin earned his PhD in special education from the University of Illinois, with a focus on transition. He taught for 2 years at Eastern Illinois University, then became a professor at the University of Colorado at Colorado Springs for 16 years. While at Colorado he served as the special education program coordinator and was director of the Center for Self-Determination. Dr. Martin has authored several books, numerous journal articles and chapters for edited books, and several curriculum lesson packages, which include video and multimedia applications. Federal, state, and local agencies have provided funding for his research and writing activities. He has conducted presentations and training workshops at sites across the United States, Canada, and Europe. Dr. Martin's professional interests focus on the transition of youth with disabilities from high school into postsecondary education and the workforce. In particular, he is interested in the application of self-determination methodology to educational and workplace settings.

Dennis E. Mithaug, PhD, is Professor of Education in the Department of Health and Behavior Studies at Teachers College, Columbia University. He has written a number of journal articles and book chapters, and has authored, coauthored or coedited several books, including *Self-Instruction Pedagogy: How to Teach Self-Determined Learning* (2007) and *Theory in Self-Determination: Foundations for Educational Practice* (2003). Dr. Mithaug received his BA in psychology from Dartmouth College, and an MA and PhD in sociology and MEd in special education from the University of Washington.

Susan B. Palmer, PhD, is Research Associate Professor at the Beach Center on Disability at the University of Kansas. She is codeveloper of the *Self-Determined Learning Model of Instruction,* coauthor of *Whose Future Is It Anyway?,* and lead author of *A Teacher's Guide to Implementing the Self-Determined Learning Model of Instruction, Early Elementary Version.* Dr. Palmer's research interests are in the development of self-determination and early intervention to enhance future self-determination. Prior to coming to the University of Kansas, she was project director at The Arc of the United States. Dr. Palmer received her doctorate in Human Development with an emphasis on evaluation, early childhood, and disabilities from the University of Texas at Dallas, and has published and presented widely on issues pertaining to the development of self-determination and interventions to promote that outcome. In 2003 she received the Distinguished Researcher Award from Region V of the American Association on Mental Retardation (AAMR). She has served as president of the Kansas chapter of the AAMR, as well as president of its education division.

Series Editors' Note

Making choices and expressing preferences are a critical part of the human experience. Only recently, however, have researchers and practitioners begun to come together to focus on how individuals with intellectual and developmental disabilities can become more capable of making their own choices and expressing their preferences. Research indicates that implementing strategies to promote self-determination can have positive effects on behavior, learning, transition to work and community, and social relationships. In fact, federal policy now includes a focus on development of self-determination for individuals with intellectual and developmental disabilities.

Promoting Self-Determination in Students with Developmental Disabilities offers a unique and invaluable contribution to the field, at just the time that it is needed. Teachers, teacher educators, other practitioners, and families will find a wealth of information and practical approaches for the development of self-determination in this book, which is part of the What Works for Special-Needs Learners series. This series addresses the education of learners with special needs—students who are at risk, those with disabilities, and all children and adolescents who struggle with learning or behavior. Researchers in special education, educational psychology, curriculum and instruction, and other fields have made great progress in understanding what works for struggling learners, yet the practical application of this research remains quite limited. This is due in part to the lack of appropriate materials for teachers, teacher educators, and inservice teacher development programs. Books in this series present assessment, instructional, and classroom management methods with a strong research base and provide specific "how-to" instructions and examples of the use of proven procedures in schools.

Promoting Self-Determination in Students with Developmental Disabilities provides readers first with a clear and comprehensive explanation of self-determination and why it is important to students with disabilities. Next, the roles of choice making, problem solving, decision making, goal setting, and self-advocacy in promoting self-determination are explored, and concrete applications for students with intellectual and developmental disabilities are provided. In addition, the authors explain how to teach individuals with disabilities to use self-instructions, self-monitoring, self-evaluation, and cues for behavior, resulting in a model to teach students to self-regulate the learning process. They also discuss how technology and universal design can play important roles in promoting self-determination and carefully explore student involvement in educational planning.

Current books in this series have focused on the application of research to the education of students with special needs in such areas as strategy instruction for students with learning disabilities, teaching word recognition, teaching mathematics, and developing reading comprehension. Future books in this series will cover such issues as social skills instruction, working with families, academic instruction for students with behavioral and emotional difficulties, and writing. All volumes will be as thorough and detailed as the present one and will facilitate implementation of evidence-based practices in classrooms, schools, and communities.

KAREN R. HARRIS
STEVE GRAHAM

Prologue

Promoting the self-determination of children and youth with disabilities has become both an expectation of federal disability policy and a significant focus in the education of students with disabilities, particularly students with intellectual and developmental disabilities. As a result of the federal emphasis on and funding to promote self-determination as a component of the education of transition-age youth with disabilities, many resources are now available to support instruction to achieve this outcome, ranging from curricular materials and guides to instructional strategies and methods, assessment tools, teaching models, model programs, and student-directed planning programs.

Most of the evidence supporting the implementation of strategies to promote self-determination is derived from studies examining the impact of instruction to promote component elements of self-determined behavior. For example, providing opportunities for students to make choices and enhancing the capacity of youth with intellectual and developmental disabilities to express preferences have been linked to multiple outcomes of benefit to transition, including improved outcomes for community-based instruction and more positive vocational outcomes. There is an emerging knowledge base showing that incorporating choice making into interventions to reduce problem behaviors of students with disabilities results in improved behavioral outcomes.

Teaching effective decision-making and problem-solving skills also has been shown to enhance positive transition outcomes for youth and young adults with intellectual and developmental disabilities, including improving leisure skill acquisition and vocational outcomes. Limitations in social problem-solving skills have been linked to difficulties in employment, participation in the community, and independent living situations for adults with developmental disabilities, and research has found that teaching such problem-solving skills to students contributes to more positive workplace social interactions later in life. Further, research shows that teaching students with intellectual and developmental disabilities to self-regulate the problem-solving process enables them to self-direct learning and to achieve educationally relevant goals, including goals linked to state and local standards.

Similarly, research links enhanced self-management and self-regulation skills to the attainment of positive adult outcomes for youth with intellectual and developmental disabilities. Teaching students self-monitoring strategies has been shown to improve critical learning skills and classroom involvement skills of students with severe disabilities. Likewise, teaching students with intellectual and developmental disabilities goal-setting, self-monitoring, and self-evaluation strategies improved work productivity.

Research on these component elements of self-determined behavior provides strong, though indirect, evidence that students with intellectual and developmental disabilities who are more self-determined achieve more positive adult outcomes. There are also a few studies that provide direct evidence of the relationship between self-determination and positive transition outcomes, including more positive employment, independent living, and community participation outcomes.

In summary, an expanding base of evidence suggests that a higher level of self-determination and increased capacity in the component elements of self-determined behavior result in better education-related outcomes for youth with disabilities. The purpose of this book is to provide a comprehensive review of what works in promoting the self-determination of children and youth with intellectual and developmental disabilities; to introduce teachers working with this population to self-determination; and to familiarize these teachers with empirically validated practices to promote self-determination, its component elements, and self-determined learning. Our aim is not to cover every existing program, curriculum, or strategy but to identify those instructional programs or methodologies that have an empirical basis. We approach this task with the intent that promoting self-determination should not be a separate, stand-alone curricular area but that such efforts should be infused into the general education curriculum and conducted in the context of the general education classroom.

The book is organized into four main sections. Part I provides a comprehensive overview of the self-determination construct; its applicability to and impact on the education of students with disabilities, particularly students with intellectual and developmental disabilities; and the role of student-directed learning in quality educational supports for this population. Part II focuses on promoting self-determined behavior, and chapters in this section explore the component elements of choice making, problem solving, decision making, goal setting, and self-advocacy and identify instructional strategies to promote this outcome. Part III covers student-directed learning strategies that enable students to become more self-determined, including antecedent event regulation strategies, such as picture cues; consequent event regulation strategies, such as self-monitoring and self-evaluation; and self-instruction. This section concludes with a chapter introducing a combination of these strategies into a model to teach students to self-regulate the learning process. Part IV discusses practices to promote student involvement in educational planning and decision making and the role of technology and universal design for learning in students' educational programs.

In this book we use the term "intellectual and developmental disabilities" to describe the students for whom these practices will be implemented. Neither intellectual nor developmental disabilities are Individuals with Disabilities Education Act (IDEA) categorical areas determining eligibility for special education services. In general, the methods, materials, and practices covered in this book have been validated with students receiving special education services under the categories of mental retardation, multiple disabilities, other health impairments, autism, and orthopedic impairments. Most of the instructional strategies and methods discussed, however, have not been developed either categorically or as condition specific. The term "intellectual and developmental disabilities," then, is a means to refer to a broader array of student support needs than those identified by either an IDEA category or a specific medical or psychological condition or diagnosis.

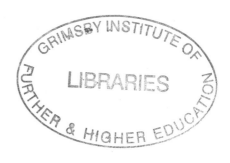
Contents

PART IV. CURRICULUM MODIFICATIONS AND STUDENT INVOLVEMENT

PART I

INTRODUCTION

CHAPTER 1

Overview of Self-Determination and Self-Determined Learning

Promoting self-determination has become best practice in the education of students with disabilities. One example corroborating this statement is the 2003 report of the President's Commission on Excellence in Special Education, which stated:

> While the Commission wholeheartedly supports strong academic achievement for all students, it recognizes that academic achievement alone will not lead to successful results for students with disabilities. Students with disabilities need educational supports and services to promote the acquisition of skills throughout their school lives. However, these supports and services may need to intensify during the transition years. Such skills include self-determination, self-advocacy, social skills, organizational skills, community and peer connection, communication, conflict resolution, career skill building and career development and computer/technological competency. (p. 47)

With all due respect to the President's Commission, in this book we choose not to categorize efforts to promote self-determination as a separate set of skills important to one type of educational outcome, whether academic achievement, employment, interpersonal relationships, or community inclusion. While traditionally classified as a focus of transition services, and thus more frequently linked to transition services mandated by the Individuals with Disabilities Education Act (IDEA), promoting the self-determination of children and youth with and without intellectual and developmental disabilities has implications across the lifespan and across life domains. Though most interventions have been developed and validated with middle and high school students, promoting the outcome that students leave school as self-determined young people is a lifelong focus for families and educators.

It is critical to establish what we mean when we use the term "self-determination." While the remaining chapters focus on interventions to promote self-determination, this chapter provides a theoretically based discussion of the term's history and usage to clarify and specify what it means. This is important because "self-determination" is a construct—a disposition or characteristic of a person that, hypothetically, helps explain and predict some aspect of his or her behavior. Self-determination cannot be directly observed, only inferred from proxy behaviors, actions, or reports; it cannot be measured directly, like weight or temperature, but must be estimated from these proxy behaviors and actions, from self-reports about the intent of these actions, and from perceptions about them. The educational use of this construct is derived most directly from its use in psychology; though, as discussed subsequently, that field inherited the construct from the discipline of philosophy, and its understanding in both psychology and education derive from this earliest use.

WHAT IS SELF-DETERMINATION?

We cannot teach children to become more self-determined until we know what it means to be self-determined. The *Oxford English Dictionary* (Simpson & Weiner, 1989) identified the earliest use of *self-determination* as occurring in 1683 and defines it as referring to the "determination of one's mind or will by itself toward an object" (p. 919). Similarly, the *American Heritage Dictionary of the English Language* (1992) defined *self-determination* as the "determination of one's own fate or course of action without compulsion; free will." As these definitions indicate, the term pertains at its basic level to issues of human action as a function of mind, will, and/or volition.

To understand the intent of the self-determination construct as used today, one must begin with an examination of issues pertaining to determinism. (See Wehmeyer, Abery, Mithaug, and Stancliffe [2003], from which the following discussion has been summarized, for a more extensive discussion of theoretical foundations of self-determination.) "Determinism" is the philosophical doctrine positing that events (in this context, human behavior) are effects of preceding causes.

Self-Determination in Psychology

The most recent and widespread use of self-determination as a psychological construct appears in the research of psychologists Edward Deci and Richard Ryan (Deci & Ryan, 1985, 2003), who proposed a theory of intrinsic motivation that incorporated a central role for self-determination. Deci and Ryan (Deci, 1975; Deci & Ryan, 1985) proposed that people have an intrinsic need to be self-determining and proposed their Self-Determination Theory as "distinguish[ing] between the motivational dynamics underlying activities that people do freely and those that they feel coerced or pressured to do. To be self-determining means to engage in an activity with a full sense of wanting, choosing, and personal endorsement. When self-determined, people are acting in accord with, or expressing, themselves" (Deci, 1992, p. 44). Within Self-Determination Theory, Deci and Ryan (1985) define self-determination as

> the capacity to choose and to have those choices, rather than reinforcement contingencies, drives, or any other forces or pressures, to be the determinants of one's actions. But self-determination is *more than a capacity, it is also a need* [italics added]. We have posited a basic, innate propensity to be self-determining that leads organisms to engage in interesting behaviors. (p. 38)

DEFINING SELF-DETERMINATION

Self-determination is a psychological construct applied to an educational context, and it implies that individuals (e.g., selves) *cause* themselves to act in certain ways, as opposed to someone or something causing them to act in certain other ways (Mithaug, 1998). This self–other dichotomy is not equivalent to saying that self-determination refers to actions caused by forces internal to the person versus forces external to the person because obviously genes, neurotransmitters, and other determinants of human behavior are internal to the person. Instead, the use of the self-determinism construct is linked to the capacity of humans to override other determinants or causes of their behavior so as to act based on their own will or volition. Self-determination refers, then, to volitional actions, where "volition" refers to making conscious *choices* or the power or will to make conscious choices.

"Conscious" is defined as intentionally conceived or done, or deliberate. "Volitional behavior" implies that one acts consciously, with intent, and "intentional action" refers to actions done deliberately and purposefully. Self-determined behavior is volitional and intentional, not random and nonpurposeful.

THEORIES OF SELF-DETERMINATION

The self-determination construct was first widely applied to the context of the education of students with disabilities in the early 1990s as an outcome of then newly introduced federal mandates pertaining to transition services and student involvement in transition planning. Since that time, several theoretical frameworks have emerged to define self-determination and operationalize it within the context of special education services. This book draws on two of these theoretical frameworks, described briefly here.

A Functional Theory of Self-Determination

Wehmeyer and colleagues (Wehmeyer, 2001, 2006) proposed a functional theory of self-determination, so called because it emphasizes that self-determination must be defined and self-determined behaviors identified by the function they serve for the individual. Accordingly, within this theoretical framework, "self-determination refers to volitional actions that enable one to act as the primary causal agent in one's life and to maintain or improve one's quality of life" (Wehmeyer, 2006, p. 117). The volitional actions defining self-determination are characterized as having four *essential characteristics*: (1) the person acted *autonomously*; (2) the behavior was *self-regulated*; (3) the person initiated and responded to the event in a *psychologically empowered* manner; and (4) the person acted in a *self-realizing* manner. These characteristics describe the *function* of the behavior that makes it self-determined or not. The model is depicted graphically in Figure 1.1, and greater detail on the essential elements of self-determined behaviors is available in Wehmeyer, Abery, and colleagues (2003).

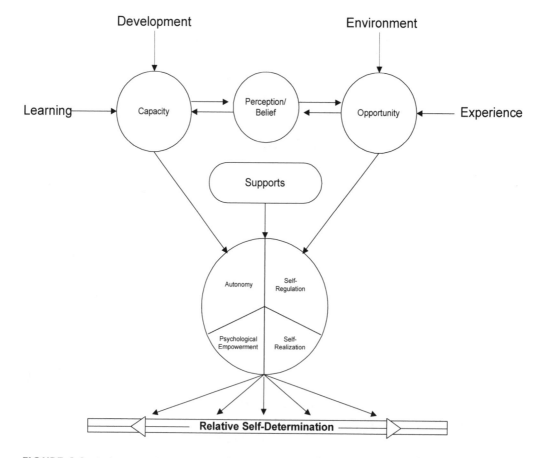

FIGURE 1.1. A functional model of self-determination. From Wehmeyer, Agran, and Hughes (1998). Copyright 1998 by Michael Wehmeyer, Martin Agran, and Carolyn Hughes. Reprinted by permission.

At the heart of this definition is the notion of causal agency. The adjective "causal" is defined as expressing or indicating cause, showing the interaction of cause and effect. The term "agent" means one who acts or has the authority to act or, alternatively, a force or substance that causes change. Self-determined people are "causal agents" in their own lives. They act with authority to make or cause things to happen in their lives. Causal agency implies more, however, than just causing action. It implies that the individual who causes things to happen in his or her life does so with an eye toward accomplishing a specific end or causing change; in other words, the individual acts volitionally and intentionally. Causal agency, as opposed to implying only that an individual caused an event to happen, implies that an action was purposeful or performed to achieve an end. Bandura (1997) noted:

> People can exercise influence over what they do. Most human behavior, of course, is determined by many interacting factors, and so people are contributors to, rather than the sole determiners of, what happens to them. In evaluating the role of intentionality in human agency, one must distinguish between the personal production of action for an intended outcome and the effects that carrying out that course of action actually produce. Agency refers to acts done intentionally. (p. 3)

People who consistently engage in self-determined behaviors can be described as self-determined, where *self-determined* refers to a "dispositional characteristic." Dispositional characteristics involve the organization of cognitive, psychological, and physiological elements in such a manner that an individual's behavior in different situations will be similar. Eder (1990) described dispositional states as frequent, enduring tendencies used to characterize people and describe important differences between people. As such, people can be described as self-determined based on the functional characteristics of their actions or behaviors.

Self-determination emerges across the lifespan as children and adolescents learn skills and develop attitudes that enable them to become causal agents in their own lives. These attitudes and abilities are the component elements of self-determination, and it is this level of the theoretical framework that drives instructional activities. The essential characteristics that define self-determined behavior emerge through the development and acquisition of these multiple, interrelated component elements. Although Table 1.1 is not intended as an exhaustive taxonomy, the component elements it lists are important to the emergence of self-determined behavior.

Each component element is addressed in a chapter of this book. In addition to providing a level at which intervention can occur, each of these component elements has a unique developmental course or is acquired through specific learning experiences, and by describing the development of each of these component elements, we can describe the development of self-determination (Doll, Sands, Wehmeyer, & Palmer, 1996; Wehmeyer, Sands, Doll, & Palmer, 1997). The development and acquisition of these component elements is lifelong. Some elements have

TABLE 1.1. Component Elements of Self-Determined Behavior

- Choice-making skills
- Decision-making skills
- Problem-solving skills
- Goal-setting and attainment skills
- Independence, risk-taking, and safety skills
- Self-observation, evaluation, and reinforcement skills
- Self-instruction skills
- Self-advocacy and leadership skills
  - Positive attributions of efficacy and outcome expectancy
  - Self-awareness
  - Self-knowledge

greater applicability for secondary education and transition, while others are more important in the elementary years. Promoting self-determination as an educational outcome requires not only a purposeful instructional program, but also one that coordinates learning experiences across the span of a student's educational experience.

Empirical Validation of the Functional Model

This theoretical model was initially derived from focus groups of people with intellectual and developmental disabilities (Wehmeyer, 1992a) and a comprehensive review of the pertinent literature (Wehmeyer, 1992b). To test the theory, Wehmeyer, Kelchner, and Richards (1996) conducted a series of structured interviews with individuals with mental retardation in order to examine the contribution of essential characteristics of self-determined behavior to the achievement of behavioral outcomes closely associated with self-determination. These interviews were conducted with more than 400 adults with mental retardation using self-report measures of self-determined behavior (Wehmeyer, Kelchner, & Richards, 1995) and measures of each of the essential characteristics (Wehmeyer et al., 1996). Upon completion of data collection activities, the sample was divided into two groups, those who scored high on the self-report measure and those who scored low. These groups were compared based on their self-determination scores on measures of each essential characteristic. Scores from measures of each of the four essential characteristics differed significantly based on self-determination group. In each case, individuals who were in the high-self-determination group held more positive beliefs or exhibited more adaptive behaviors. In essence, the study indicated that each of the four essential characteristics was predictive of self-determination status. Measures of behavioral autonomy and self-regulation were particularly potent predictors of self-determination status.

SELF-DETERMINATION AS SELF-REGULATED PROBLEM SOLVING

Mithaug, Campeau, and Wolman (1992) suggested that "self-determination is a special form of self-regulation—one that is unusually effective and markedly free of external influence" (p. 4), in which people who are self-determined regulate their choices and actions more successfully than people who are not. Mithaug (e.g., 1991, 1993, 1996a, 1996b, 1998) has described a model of self-determination as self-regulated problem solving. Mithaug (1993) suggested that individuals are often in flux between existing states and goals or desired states. When a discrepancy exists between what one has and what one wants, an incentive for self-regulation and subsequent action may be operative. With the realization that a problem or discrepancy exists, the individual may set out to achieve the goal or desired state. Because of a history of failure or a sense of powerlessness or learned helplessness, individuals with disabilities may do little to change their situations. They may set expectations that are too low or, in some cases, too high. As Mithaug (1993) noted, negative feelings produce low expectations. Inaccurate self-assessments may produce unrealistic or unfeasible expectations.

To promote success, individuals need to enhance or increase their expectations. The ability to set appropriate expectations is based on the individual's success in matching his or her capacity with present opportunity. "Capacity" is the individual's assessment of existing resources (e.g., skills, interests, motivation), and "opportunity" refers to the aspects of the existing situation that will allow him or her to achieve the desired goal. Mithaug referred to optimal prospects as "just-right" matches in which individuals are able to correctly match their capacities with existing opportunities. The experience generated during self-regulation "is a function of repeated interaction between capacity and opportunity over time" (Mithaug, 1996a, p. 159). As Mithaug (1996a) noted, "the more competent we are, the fewer errors we make, and the less time we take, the greater the gain we produce" (p. 156).

Mithaug (1993) summarized self-regulation theory as stating that "we maximize progress toward goals when (1) past gains match expectations, (2) present expectations are the maximum possible, (3) choices are the best possible, and (4) follow-through on choice is as effective and efficient as possible" (p. 60). Such circumstances optimize adjustment to maximize gain for the individual. Self-determination is a "variant of self-regulated behavior" (Mithaug, 1993, p. 61) that "involves self-regulated problem solving to get what you need and want in life" (Mithaug, Wehmeyer, Agran, Martin, & Palmer, 1998). Mithaug et al. (1998) described self-determination as

> solving a *sequence of problems* in order to construct a means–end chain—a causal sequence—that moves us from where we are—an actual state of not having our needs and interests satisfied—to where we want to be—a goal state of having those needs and interests satisfied. It [e.g., self-determination] is problem solving to reduce or eliminate this discrepancy between what we want and what we have. (p. 303)

According to this analysis, "self-determination is more than solving one prob-lem in order to get what one needs and wants in life. It is solving many problems that are connected in a means–ends chain or chains. Consequently, it requires the regulation of many problem solving activities to connect needs and wants with actions and results" (Mithaug et al., 1998, pp. 303–304).

Mithaug (1998) noted that "self-determination always occurs in a social con-text" and suggested that the social nature of the concept is worth reviewing because the "distinction between self-determination and other-determination is nearly always in play when assessing an individual's prospects for controlling [his or her] life in a particular situation" (p. 42).

What Is Self-Determined Learning?

These theoretical frameworks emphasize the role of the person as a causal agent in his or her life or in self-regulating problem solving. As such, interventions derived from both models to promote self-determination have embraced the importance of student-directed learning as a means to achieve self-determined learning. Agran, King-Sears, Wehmeyer, and Copeland (2003) defined "student-directed learning" as teaching students strategies that enable them to modify and regulate their own behavior and to direct their own learning. Student-directed means that the student is an active participant in the instructional process and, to the maximum extent possible, responsible for his or her educational goal attainment. As discussed in Chapters 6–9, self-determined learning involves students choosing learning tasks and goals and adjusting goals and plans as a function of their involvement with and evaluation of their progress.

Is Self-Determination Important to Students with Intellectual and Developmental Disabilities?

An emerging special education literature base reports that promoting self-determination is a valued and important outcome for students with disabilities, including students with intellectual and developmental disabilities, but that too many of these students are not self-determined (Wehmeyer, 2006). Although a com-prehensive review of those research findings is beyond the scope of this chapter, sufficient data document limited self-determination (Stancliffe, Abery, & Smith, 2000; Wehmeyer et al., 1995; Wehmeyer & Metzler, 1995) and that students with disabilities have limited opportunities to learn skills related to self-determination (Stancliffe, 1997; Stancliffe & Abery, 1997; Stancliffe et al., 2000; Stancliffe & Wehmeyer, 1995; Wehmeyer et al., 1995).

A recent meta-analysis showed that students with disabilities benefit from in-struction to promote self-determination (Algozzine, Browder, Karvonen, Test, & Wood, 2001). Algozzine and colleagues searched the disability-related literature for articles reporting empirical evaluations of any effort to promote a component ele-ment of self-determined behavior. Fifty-one articles from 1978 to 2000 were identified, 9 of which met the criteria for inclusion in a group-design meta-analysis and 14 of which met the criteria for a single-subject–design meta-analysis. The group-design meta-analysis indicated that the studies included showed moderate gains as a result of interventions to promote a component element of self-determined behavior. The single-subject–design meta-analysis also showed that these interventions were moderately effective. In essence, there is evidence that students with disabilities can learn component elements of self-determined behavior.

That they appear to have relatively few opportunities to do so is a problem if, in fact, enhanced self-determination leads to more positive outcomes. The hypothesis that self-determination is important for more positive outcomes is supported by the literature when one examines the contributions of component elements of self-determined behavior to more favorable school and adult outcomes and studies that tested this hypothesis directly. A comprehensive review of the impact of component elements of self-determined behavior on outcomes is beyond the scope of this chapter (and each element will be addressed in a subsequent chapter), but a brief overview of the evidence that such an instructional focus can result in more positive functional and academic outcomes for students with intellectual and developmental disabilities seems warranted.

For example, providing opportunities for choice making and enhancing the capacity of youth and young adults with disabilities to express preferences have been linked to several positive outcomes. An emerging literature base shows that incorporating choice-making opportunities into interventions to reduce problem behaviors of children and youth with disabilities results in improved behavioral outcomes (Shogren, Faggella-Luby, Bae, & Wehmeyer, 2004). Cooper and Browder (1998) found that teaching young adults with intellectual disabilities to make choices improved outcomes of community-based instruction. Watanabe and Sturmey (2003) found that promoting choice-making opportunities in vocational tasks for young adults with intellectual disabilities increased engagement in the tasks.

Teaching effective decision-making and problem-solving skills also has been shown to enhance positive transition outcomes for youth and young adults with disabilities. Teaching young women with intellectual disabilities to make more effective decisions improved their capacity to identify potentially abusive social interactions (Khemka, 2000). Datillo and Hoge (1999) found that teaching adolescents with intellectual disabilities decision making in the context of a leisure education program improved their acquisition of socially valid leisure knowledge and skills.

Limitations in social problem-solving skills have been linked to difficulties in employment, community, and independent living situations for persons with intellectual and developmental disabilities (Gumpel, Tappe, & Araki, 2000). Storey (2002) reviewed the empirical literature pertaining to improving social interactions for workers with disabilities, and determined that problem-solving skills contributed to more positive workplace social interactions. O'Reilly, Lancioni, and O'Kane (2000) found that incorporating instruction in problem solving into social skills instruction improved employment outcomes for supported workers with disabilities. Finally, in Chapter 9, several studies (Agran, Blanchard, & Wehmeyer, 2000; Palmer, Wehmeyer, Gipson, & Agran, 2004; Wehmeyer, Palmer, Agran, Mithaug, & Martin, 2000) show that teaching students with disabilities a self-regulated problem-solving process enables them to self-direct learning and to achieve educationally relevant goals, including transition-related goals.

Similarly, research links enhanced self-management and self-regulation skills to the attainment of positive adult outcomes. Teaching students self-monitoring strategies has been shown to improve critical learning skills and classroom involvement skills of students with severe disabilities (Agran et al., 2005; Gilberts, Agran, Hughes, & Wehmeyer, 2001; Hughes et al., 2002). Grossi and Heward (1998) showed that teaching young adults with developmental disabilities goal-setting, self-monitoring, and self-evaluation strategies improved their work productivity. Browder and Minarovic (2000) taught workers with intellectual disabilities self-instruction strategies for job tasks in work environments, resulting in enhanced performance and employer satisfaction. Woods and Martin (2004) found that teaching supported employees to self-regulate work tasks improved employers' perceptions of the employees and improved employees' work performance.

Research on these component elements of self-determined behavior provides strong, though indirect, evidence that youth who are more self-determined achieve more positive adult outcomes. A few studies provide direct evidence of the relationship between self-determination and positive outcomes. Wehmeyer and Schwartz (1997) measured the self-determination of 80 students with learning disabilities or mental retardation and then examined adult outcomes 1 year after high school. Students in the high self-determination group were twice as likely (80%) as youth in the low self-determination group (40%) to be employed, and earned, on average, $2.00 an hour more than students in the low self-determination group who were employed. There were no significant differences between groups in level of intelligence or number of vocational courses taken. Wehmeyer and Palmer (2003) conducted a second follow-up study, examining adult status of 94 students with cognitive disabilities 1 and 3 years post-graduation. One year after high school, students in the high self-determination group were disproportionately likely to have moved from where they were living during high school, and by the third year they were still disproportionately likely to live somewhere other than their high school home and were significantly more likely than students in the low self-determination group to live independently. For employed students, those scoring higher in self-determination made statistically significant advances in obtaining job benefits, including vacation, sick leave, and health insurance, an outcome not shared by their peers in the low self-determination group.

Sowers and Powers (1995) showed that students with disabilities involved in instruction to promote self-determination increased their participation and independence in performing community activities. Finally, Wehmeyer and Schwartz (1998) examined the link between self-determination and quality of life for 50 adults with intellectual disabilities. Controlling for level of intelligence and environmental factors, they found that self-determination predicted group membership based on quality-of-life scores. That is, adults who were highly self-determined experienced a higher quality of life; adults who lacked self-determination appeared to experience a less positive quality of life.

In summary, an expanding base of evidence suggests that higher self-determination and increased capacity in the component elements of self-determined behavior result in better outcomes for youth and young adults with disabilities.

SELF-DETERMINATION AND ACCESS
TO THE GENERAL EDUCATION CURRICULUM

As noted, most of the emphasis on promoting self-determination has been on the benefit to student attainment of functional outcomes, such as employment and community inclusion. It is evident, however, that within the context of current educational reform efforts the emphasis is on student academic achievement, particularly in core academic areas such as literacy, math, and science. We believe it is important to contextualize efforts to promote self-determination not as distinct from, but within, instructional efforts to promote student access to and progress in the general education curriculum. As noted at the start of this chapter, promoting self-determination is important across the lifespan and across educational and life domains.

Wehmeyer, Field, Doren, Jones, and Mason (2004) identified two ways that promoting self-determination can enhance access to the general curriculum. First, virtually every set of state-adopted standards contains achievement standards students are expected to meet by learning and applying effective problem-solving, decision-making, and goal-setting skills. By identifying where in the general education curriculum all students are expected to learn skills and knowledge related to the component elements of self-determined behavior, teachers can promote self-determination and access to the general education curriculum.

Second, teaching students with disabilities the skills they need to become more self-determined, such as problem-solving, goal-setting, and decision-making skills, and enabling them to self-direct learning provides them with valuable skills to enhance their academic performance. Kame'enui and Simmons (1999) identified one basic design principle of curriculum adaptation as the use of "conspicuous strategies," noting,

> [t]o solve problems, students follow a set of steps or strategies. Many students develop their own strategies, but a considerable amount of time may be required for the student to identify the optimum strategy. For students with disabilities, such an approach is highly problematic because instructional time is a precious commodity and these learners may never figure out an efficient strategy. Learning is most efficient when a teacher can make it conspicuous or explicit. (p. 15)

Students who learn effectively set learning goals and objectives to reach those goals, then use problem-solving and self-regulation skills to tackle activities to achieve those goals, all components of instruction to promote self-determination.

Preliminary support for promoting self-determination with students with intellectual and developmental disabilities exists in two ways. First, multiple studies confirm that student-directed learning strategies can be taught to enable students with intellectual and developmental disabilities to self-direct learning in the general education classroom (Agran, Blanchard, Hughes, & Wehmeyer, 2002; Agran et al., 2005; Copeland, Hughes, Agran, Wehmeyer, & Fowler, 2002; Gilberts et al., 2001; Hughes et al., 2002; Wehmeyer, Hughes, Agran, Garner & Yeager, 2003; Wehmeyer, Yeager, Wade, Agran, & Hughes, 2003).

Second, two studies have tested the impact of interventions to promote self-determination on student progress toward goals derived from the general education curriculum. Palmer and colleagues (2004) examined the attainment of goals linked to science, social studies, or language arts standards for 22 middle school students with intellectual disabilities. Students learned to self-direct learning to address a goal that was derived from the state standard in each content area and that emphasized a self-determination focus. Students achieved educationally relevant goals tied to district-level standards at expected or greater than expected levels, supporting the hypothesis that instruction in self-determination can serve as an entry point to the general curriculum for students with disabilities. Similarly, Agran, Cavin, Wehmeyer, and Palmer (2006) conducted a single-subject–design study providing evidence that students with intellectual disabilities could acquire skills linked to goals in the general curriculum.

SUMMARY

Self-determination refers to people acting volitionally and intentionally to become causal agents in their own lives. There is clear evidence that enabling students with disabilities to become self-determined is linked to more positive functional outcomes. There is preliminary evidence that promoting self-determination can also promote student access to and progress in the general education curriculum, but there is also evidence that the presence of an intellectual disability or a severe disability in students limits the degree to which educators focus on promoting self-determination as an educational outcome (Wehmeyer, Agran, & Hughes, 2000). The purpose of this text is to provide a comprehensive review of what works in promoting the self-determination of children and youth with intellectual and developmental disabilities. The remaining chapters are intended to familiarize teachers working with students with intellectual and developmental disabilities with empirically validated practices to promote self-determination and its component elements.

PART II

PROMOTING SELF-DETERMINATION

CHAPTER 2

Assessing Preferences
and Promoting Choice Making

Making choices and expressing preferences are often associated with self-determination, and choice making is the component element most frequently addressed in the literature, particularly pertaining to students with severe disabilities (Martin, Valenzuela, Woods, & Borland, 2004; Wehmeyer, Agran, & Hughes, 2000; Wood, Fowler, Uphold, & Test, 2005). Like all people, people with intellectual and developmental disabilities have preferences (Cannella, O'Reilly, & Lancioni, 2005; Hagopian, Long, & Rush, 2004). Some people prefer pineapple rather than mushrooms on their pizza; some would rather work in a quiet, undisturbed setting than in a lively, dynamic environment; some would rather follow than take the lead on a task. Making choices in our lives is an activity most of us take for granted. Students with intellectual and developmental disabilities, however, too often have had limited opportunities to make choices and decisions based on their own preferences and little choice in relation to the events that affect their everyday lives (Romaniuk & Miltenberger, 2001; Shevin & Klein, 1984).

This lack of opportunities to make everyday choices or express preferences typically results in limited development of choice-making skills for students with disabilities (Cannella et al., 2005). Shevin and Klein (1984) called for creating opportunities to enable students and adults with intellectual and developmental disabilities to make choices but warned that this would be done in "relatively uncharted territory, without the comforts of traditional behavioral definitions and research methodologies" (p. 161). Fortunately, since this admonition, the field has learned much about promoting choice making. Making choices in one's life is a basic human right and a part of typical development that benefits both the person and society (Martin, Woods, Sylvester, & Gardner, 2005; Martin, Mithaug, Oliphant, Husch, & Frazier, 2002; Romaniuk & Miltenberger, 2001). The Individuals with Disabilities Education Act (IDEA; 1990), in fact, requires that transition services be based on students' interests and preferences (Johnson, 2005).

Research suggests that there are too few opportunities for students to make choices and that teachers do not believe they are equipped to teach choice making to students (Agran, Hughes, & Washington, 2006; Mason, Field, & Sawilowsky, 2004; Mithaug, 2005; Wehmeyer et al., 2000). Teaching choice making requires that systematic, structured opportunities to choose that incorporate individual preferences be embedded into students' everyday schedules (Lohrmann-O'Rourke & Gomez, 2001). While choice opportunities happen naturally for most people, the literature suggests that structured intervention strategies must be used to establish choice opportunities for students with intellectual and developmental disabilities (Lancioni, O'Reilly, & Emerson, 1996). Students must be allowed to act on their choices and experience the natural consequences of those choices (Agran & Hughes, 2005). Further, opportunities to choose must extend beyond immediate, everyday choices, such as what to wear or eat, to long-term lifestyle choices, such as where or with whom to live or whether to attend college or go to work (Bambara, 2004; Lohrmann-O'Rourke & Gomez, 2001).

For students with intellectual and developmental disabilities, multiple barriers to opportunities to choose often exist. Others too often presume that these students have few preferences, so their opportunities to choose or express preferences may be severely restricted. Further, because of these students' perceived lack of choice-making ability, others may make choices for them because they think they know best (Mithaug, 2005). Students with more severe disabilities do not express their preferences through conventional means, and, consequently, their choices may not be recognized or acknowledged (Cannella et al., 2005; Lattimore, Parsons, & Reid, 2003). For example, a student may act out to avoid performing a task he or she dislikes rather than ask to be given a break from it. By acting out, a student is expressing a preference, but others may not recognize such behavior as an expression of preference (Kern, Mantegna, Vorndran, Bailin, & Hilt, 2001; Lohrmann-O'Rourke, Browder, & Brown, 2000). Research shows that as choice-making opportunities increase, instances of problem behavior decrease (Cannella et al., 2005; Morgan, 2006). Educators must also be aware of and responsive to a student's cultural background, such as ethnicity, family-held values or beliefs, socioeconomic status, or sexual orientation, that may influence his or her preferences or manner of expressing these preferences (Agran & Hughes, 2005; Valenzuela & Martin, 2005; Zhang, 2005).

If students do not learn to make choices based on their own interests and to experience and learn from the consequences of these choices in the structured environment of the school, it is unlikely that they will be able to do so in response to the ever-changing demands of home, community, and work (Hughes, Pitkin, & Lorden, 1998). Adults may believe they are protecting students by preventing them from experiencing the consequences of poor choices (Harchik, Sherman, Sheldon,

& Bannerman, 1993; Perske, 1972; Ward, 2005, but they may actually be hindering students from learning the skills necessary to make healthy, effective decisions and the behaviors that are associated with success in employment and the community (Agran, Cain, & Cavin, 2002; Cooper & Browder, 1998).

The starting point for promoting self-determination is to provide opportunities for students with disabilities to express preferences and make choices. Explicit instruction in choice making may not be necessary for all students, but for students for whom it is necessary, it is a crucial first step to enhancing self-determination. This chapter defines choice making, gives an overview of its importance for promoting self-determination, and introduces strategies and methods to assess preferences of students who have limited communication skills. The chapter will also provide empirically validated, practical applications to infuse choice-making opportunities into the daily school routine and to teach students with more severe disabilities appropriate choice-making skills.

DEFINITION AND CONCEPTUAL BASIS OF CHOICE MAKING

The choice-making process can be conceptualized as having two distinct components: (1) a person's identification of a preference and (2) the act of choosing (Parsons, Reid, & Green, 2001; Reid, Parsons, & Green, 1991). A "preferred activity" is one that a person selects or chooses over time from several options; "choice" is the act of selecting an activity from several options with which a person is familiar (Romaniuk & Miltenberger, 2001). Choice making requires that a person be familiar and has had experience with available options, can choose without coercion, and can express a preference to others. Over time, a person develops preferences for one or more options over others.

Typically, people express preferences verbally, but the preferences of people with intellectual disabilities and/or limited communication skills must often be inferred from the act of choosing. People, places, or things that are chosen consistently over time typically are preferred and more highly valued by an individual than other options (Logan & Gast, 2001; Lohrmann-O'Rourke & Browder, 1998). Repeatedly collecting choice outcome data over time will yield a valid and reliable preference or interest assessment (Martin et al., 2002).

IMPORTANCE OF EXPRESSING PREFERENCES
AND MAKING CHOICES

Promoting choice making is important for a number of reasons. Expressing preferences and making choices are embodied in the principle of normalization (Nirje, 1972), the concept of quality of life (Schalock, 1996; Schalock et al., 2005), the construct of self-determination (Martin, Valenzuela, et al., 2004; Mithaug, 2005; Wehmeyer, 2005), and the principle of supports (Thompson et al., 2004). Edgerton

(1988) advised that "[o]ur culture makes the right to choose for oneself a fundamental value. The right—and the necessity—to make crucial choices about one's life must be a central definition of normalization" (p. 332).

The opportunity to express one's preferences and make choices has been conceptualized as critical to building individual capacity, optimizing learning, and achieving personal growth and self-determination (Mithaug, Mithaug, Agran, Martin, & Wehmeyer, 2003). Mithaug and colleagues (2003) argued that when people with disabilities are provided opportunities to make choices and act on them, they become actively engaged in their learning process, allowing them to set goals, plan action, and make adjustments as needed.

Incorporating opportunities to choose into the daily lives of students with intellectual and developmental disabilities has been related to positive outcomes, such as increased task engagement and reduced problem behavior (Cannella et al., 2005). For example, Taber-Doughty (2005) found that when students with intellectual disabilities were given a choice of instructional methods, independent task performance and task duration increased. In addition, expressing preferences and choice making have been related to increased motivation (Foster-Johnson, Ferro, & Dunlap, 1994), academic gains (Cooper et al., 1992), increased productivity (Lancioni, O'Reilly, & Oliva, 2002), community job longevity (Martin et al., 2003), and reductions in aggressive behavior (Seybert, Dunlap, & Ferro, 1996). Providing access to preferred items, events, or situations has also been shown to have positive effects on individuals' educational performance (Kennedy & Haring, 1993; Parsons, Reid, Reynolds, & Bumgarner, 1990). Research has shown that when people with intellectual disabilities are assigned preferred rather than nonpreferred tasks, their productivity and on-task behavior increased on small-assembly jobs (Parsons et al., 1990) and that individuals adjust their choices to complete preferred tasks (Mithaug & Mar, 1980).

Despite philosophical, legislative, and empirical support for the critical role of preference and choice in improving performance, quality of life, and participation in everyday experiences, numerous studies indicate that people with intellectual and developmental disabilities have restricted opportunities to express preferences or make choices in their daily lives (Stancliffe & Wehmeyer, 1995; Wehmeyer & Metzler, 1995). Too often their everyday choices such as what to wear or eat or how to spend free time and their long-term programmatic goals such as employment are made by others. Stancliffe and Wehmeyer (1995) found that adults with intellectual disabilities had limited opportunities to choose their roommates, where they lived or worked, or what they did during their leisure time.

When one considers that studies indicate that adult caregivers' opinions of the preferences of people with intellectual and developmental disabilities frequently do not agree with those individuals' actual preferences (Lohrmann-O'Rourke & Browder, 1998; Martin et al., 2005), it is critical that people with disabilities have the opportunity to express their own preferences and make their own choices. It is particularly important (and mandated by law) that students' preferences and interests be incorporated into the transition goals of their Individualized Education Programs (IEPs). Likewise, basing job placements on an individual's preferences and choices when developing a match between a worker and a potential job has been associated with enhanced employee satisfaction and performance on the job (Martin et al., 2002).

Until recently, little research was available to guide teachers, parents, and caregivers in assessing students' preferences or providing opportunities for choice making within students' educational programming and daily activities. Wehmeyer and colleagues (2000) found that teachers felt unqualified to teach choice making. Fortunately, methods have been designed to assess the preferences of students with disabilities and teach choice-making skills. Studies indicate that caregivers and others can learn to provide opportunities for individuals to choose within their everyday lives and across environmental contexts (e.g., Browder, Cooper, & Lim, 1998).

ASSESSING PREFERENCES

Recently, several reviews of investigations of preference assessments have been conducted (Cannella et al., 2005; Hagopian et al., 2004; Hughes et al., 1998; Lohrmann-O'Rourke & Browder, 1998). Preference assessments are methods of identifying a student's preferences by systematically presenting activities or items to sample and observing the student's responses (Lohrmann-O'Rourke et al., 2000). Such procedures are particularly important for students with limited communication skills. The choice-making opportunity must be structured so that the student makes an informed choice (Martin et al., 2002), and making an informed choice relies upon the amount of practice the student has had in making choices (Rawlings, Dowse, & Shaddock, 1995). An informed vocational choice, for instance, requires direct experience with the setting, characteristics, and work tasks of the job, often over time (Schaller & Szymanski, 1992). Lohrmann-O'Rourke and Browder (1998) suggested that choice-making preference assessment for students with disabilities should include:

- Repeated opportunities for students to make choices.
- Mass trial assessment combined with observation in the actual environment where the choice exists.
- Repeated assessment across days.
- Periodic assessment across time to assess preference changes.
- Presentation of choice stimuli in a manner that students can use (e.g., actual item, picture, video clip).
- Directly selecting the choice by touching, picking up, or pointing to the chosen option.
- Presenting the choices in a paired format with limited time to make the selection.

Hanley, Iwata, and Roscoe (2006) found that preference assessment using a paired-item format produced more stable preference patterns over time than single-item preference assessment. Over time, the repeated measurement pro-

cess combined with situational assessment will yield valid and reliable preference assessment results (Martin et al., 2002; Martin, Mithaug, Husch, Frazier, &
Marshall, 2003).

In this section, we summarize findings of reviews of the preference assessment
literature, with examples from the literature to illustrate the variety of preference
assessment methods available. Because caregivers' opinions of an individual's
preferences may be inaccurate (Lohrmann-O'Rourke & Browder, 1998; Martin et
al., 2005), only studies that directly assessed preference through observation are
included. In addition, because communication skills relate directly to how an individual expresses choice or preference (Brown, Gothelf, Guess, & Lehr, 1998), only
studies that provided sufficient information to determine communication modalities of participants are included.

Assessing Students' Preference Responses

Seven methods of assessing preferences were identified. Each was based on a type
of student response: (1) use of a computer touch screen or mouse click; (2) activation of a microswitch; (3) approach toward an object; (4) verbalizations, signing,
gestures, vocalizations, or affect; (5) physical selection of an item; (6) task performance; and (7) time engaged with an item. Often, students with intellectual and
developmental disabilities, because of limited verbal or communication skills or
lack of experience or practice expressing themselves, cannot tell others what
their preferences are. Sometimes practitioners must infer preferences from a student's behavior when he or she responds to situations in which choices are presented.

Use of a Computer Touch Screen or Mouse Click Combined with Situational Assessment

An interactive multimedia vocational assessment software package titled Choose
and Take Action: Finding the Right Job for You (Martin, Marshall, Wray, et al.,
2004) uses the student-directed preference procedures advocated by Lohrmann-
O'Rourke and Browder (1998). Students who cannot read and who have little to no
previous work experience make initial job choices using the software that match
their preferred job characteristics, settings, and activities. Students choose one
video clip from each paired set depicting specific job settings, characteristics, and
activities. Each 20-second video demonstrates one of 14 commonly found employment settings, 15 entry-level activities, and 12 job characteristics. Each activity is
shown in at least two settings, and each characteristic is shown at least four times.
Then, students compare their choices to actual experiences they either observe or
have at a community job site. Students repeat this process until reliable choices
emerge that match features of specific job settings. A single-elimination process
narrows the individual's job choice, then prompts the student to choose whether he
or she wants to watch or do the identified community job. After experiencing the
job, the student evaluates his or her experiences and makes new choices based on

what he or she has learned. The software tracks and accumulates each student's choices and produces a detailed profile of his or her preferred job.

Martin and colleagues (2005) compared job choices made by high school students and adults, both with severe disabilities. Five of the participants were able to use at least one hand to access choices on a standard computer keyboard without adaptations. One participant used a single switch to indicate choices, and the remaining two verbalized or used eye gaze or an alternate gesture to make a choice (or have the researcher indicate their choice) due to inconsistent fine-motor capabilities and lack of their own assistive technology devices. Participants watched 8, 16, or 32 videos per session and decided on the job they liked best, either to watch or to do. They then watched or did their chosen job in a community setting. Educators, support staff, and caregivers ranked three settings, three activities, and three characteristics based on their perception of what they thought the individual in their care would like most.

Martin and colleagues (2005) calculated the match between the top three choices made directly by individuals with disabilities compared to the top three choices made by their caregivers. The results indicated an 18% match for top three activity choices, 33% match for top three characteristic choices, and a 36% match for top three setting choices. Next, Martin and colleagues (2005) compared the top choice made by individuals with disabilities in each category to that made on their behalf by their caregivers. The results indicated a 0% match for top activity and characteristic choices and an 18% match for the top setting choice. This study demonstrated that a small group of individuals with severe disabilities and alternative communication modalities did make distinct vocational choice that differed considerably from choices made by their caregivers.

Activation of a Microswitch

Some students with limited verbal or motor skills have difficulty expressing a preference or indicating a choice in a conventional manner. One strategy to teach students with limited use of their bodies to express preferences is to use whatever physical movement they can make to activate a microswitch to indicate a choice. Dattilo (1986) taught three students with intellectual, sensory, and motor impairments and no expressive verbal communication skills to activate microswitches that were connected to computer software. Activation of a microswitch by a slight movement of a student's body (e.g., raising arm) resulted in the activation of a choice of one of two options (indicated by, for example, video scenes, a vibrating pad, or taped music). Students' choices were tabulated automatically by the computer program. All students indicated preferences for particular items, as demonstrated by their consistently choosing these items more than others.

Approach toward an Object

Another strategy for assessing the preferences of people with a wide range of communication abilities is to observe whether they approach an object when it is presented as an option. Pace, Ivancic, Edwards, Iwata, and Page (1985) observed the responses of six students with intellectual disabilities and limited communication and adaptive skills when 16 objects were presented one at a time to each student. After each item was presented, the student's approach to the item was assessed. Ten opportunities to approach an object were presented; following an approach, the student was allowed to interact with the object. Preferred items were those that were approached in at least 80% of the presentations, and nonpreferred items were approached in 50% or fewer opportunities. All students showed definite preferences for some of the 16 items by approaching those items at least 80% of the time.

The approach strategy for assessing preferences may easily be used with any student, with or without a disability. A teacher simply needs to note, across time, which items, activities, materials, or events students tend to approach in a situation in which all choices are equally and readily available (e.g., free time).

Verbalizations, Gestures, and Affect

For students who have expressive communication skills, indications of preferences and choices may include a variety of expressive behavior, including verbalizations, manual signing, physical gestures, vocalizations, or physical affect. For example, Winking, O'Reilly, and Moon (1993) observed the expressive behavior of four employees with autism and severe behavior disorders (e.g., aggression, self-injury) as they completed a variety of jobs in a large hotel (e.g., laundry, food service, housekeeping). Observation recorded a range of behaviors for each employee that indicated preference or nonpreference of specific job tasks. For example, one young woman's preference responses included smiling, singing, and repeating certain words or sounds. Her nonpreference responses included wandering, grabbing, or crumbling materials. Employees' preference or nonpreference responses when performing various tasks in the hotel were observed in order to match employees with jobs that they liked to perform. Results from the matching showed that individuals had increased work-related skills and decreased inappropriate behavior.

Green, Gardner, and Reid (1997) found that when presented preferred options, three participants with severe intellectual disabilities had observable changes in their facial expressions indicating pleasure. This finding suggests that educators and caregivers could infer preferences by using happiness indicators. Schwartzman, Martin, Yu, and Whiteley (2004), however, were not able to replicate these findings. Participants in the second study showed very few happiness behaviors, and the degree of preference for an item had little impact on expression happiness. The conflicting results suggest that only using affect indicators may not be the most appropriate method to infer preferences.

Physical Selection of an Item

Preferences of students with intellectual and developmental disabilities can also be assessed by observing whether they physically select (e.g., pick up, circle, point, or mark) an item when it is presented. This strategy requires the item to be present in the environment, which may limit the variety of choices that can be offered. The range of options can be expanded, however, by presenting items representing an activity, event, or situation. For example, a ticket to a baseball game could represent the opportunity to see a game, a book of coupons could represent the opportunity to go grocery shopping, and illustrations or pictures could be used to facilitate choosing preferred job sites, characteristics, or tasks. Graff, Gibson, and Galiatsatos (2006) found similar preference hierarchies for adolescents with severe disabilities who responded to illustrations and those who responded to the actual items.

Martin and colleagues (2002) provided individuals with developmental disabilities job task, characteristic, and site illustrations to choose what they liked and wanted to do. Individuals would indicate their choice by pointing to the illustration or marking it. After repeating this process several times over a few days, obvious choice patterns emerged. The individual would spend time at the selected job site watching or doing the job, then choose again and again. He or she repeated this cycle of choosing, experiencing choice, and adjusting choice until a consistent, rational choice emerged—a choice that matched his or her interests and skills to an available community job. At times, actual experience at the job would change the choice profile. In an analysis of the program's data, Martin and colleagues (2003) found that future workers with developmental disabilities who completed a detailed job-matching assessment process driven by individual choice were 50% more likely to be employed and also statistically more likely to maintain a job than those who did not complete a choice assessment.

Task Performance

Another strategy for measuring preference that requires the physical presence of choice items is observing a student's performance of a specific task. Wacker, Berg, Wiggins, Muldoon, and Cavanaugh (1985) used task performance as a preference assessment strategy when they observed the performance of five students on instructional tasks (e.g., range-of-motion exercises). When the students performed a targeted behavior, they were given access to a potentially preferred item (e.g., game). Items were varied across performance sessions in order that the effect on performance of different items could be compared. Increases in task performance were associated with access to specific items. Because of the reinforcing effect these items had on task performance, they were considered to be preferred.

Time Engaged with an Item

Preference for items or activities also has been inferred from the amount of time a student continues to be engaged with a particular item in comparison to time spent with other items or activities. Kennedy and Haring (1993) used a time engagement strategy when they assessed the preferences of four students with multiple significant disabilities. Items such as a computer game or jigsaw puzzle were suggested by the students' teachers as likely either to be preferred or not preferred by each student. Subsequently, the items were placed one at a time on each student's laptop attached to his or her wheelchair, and the amount of time the student engaged with the item during 1 minute was noted and compared with time spent with other items. Engagement with an item was defined as a student physically touching the item with his or her hand or arm or facing the item. Findings showed that each student had definite preferences for interacting more with some items than with others.

Observing Students' Preference Responses over Time

In assessing a student's preferences, it is important to observe the choices a student makes over an extended period of time. The studies reviewed by Carr, Nicolson, and Higbee (2000), Hughes and colleagues (1998), and Lohrmann-O'Rourke and Browder (1998) indicated that preferences are idiosyncratic to each student. Stafford, Alberto, Fredrick, Heflin, and Heller (2002) also found that students' preferences often vary across time, which suggests the need for ongoing applied preference assessment. In addition, whereas some students tend to pick the same option for a lengthy period of time before switching to another, some vary their choices frequently. Consequently, preferences may not be evident immediately. In order to get a true picture of a student's preferences, it is important to observe and record the choices a student makes over an extended period of time. One can then estimate the percentage of times a particular option was chosen out of the total number of opportunities a student had to choose. Those options chosen a higher percentage of the time than others likely are the ones preferred by a student.

Providing Opportunities to Choose

Teachers have a variety of strategies available to provide opportunities for students to make choices and demonstrate preferences. These strategies vary according to the number and type of choices provided as well as the manner of presenting the choices.

Number of Choices

Across the reviewed studies, either one or two items or activities were provided per opportunity to choose. The number of choices presented did not vary according to the level of ability of participants. When preferences were assessed by a participant's physical selection of an item, two options were always presented. In contrast, when preferences were assessed by a participant's task performance, only one choice was offered (when one option is available, the inferred choice is whether to engage in the task or not). Across all other types of preference or choice responses, either one or two choices were presented with equally effective results in identifying preferences. Therefore, if a teacher were assessing a student's preferences by observing his or her approaches to a variety of activities or events, the teacher could present potential preferences either individually or two at a time.

A teacher also may choose to present an array of options to a student in a less controlled, more naturalistic situation. For example, Koegel, Dyer, and Bell (1987) equipped a large room with many games and toys and allowed three students with autism to choose whichever items they wished to interact with and to change to a new item as frequently as they wished. Results indicated that five preferred and nonpreferred items were identified for each student based on the amount of time he or she interacted with the items.

Type of Choices

Theoretically, the types of choices a teacher could present to students to determine their preferences are limitless. The range of options could vary from choices as simple as what to eat or wear to more complex decisions such as what classes to take, whether to accept a new job, or whom to date. In reality, empirical studies have almost exclusively assessed preferences that require fairly limited choice- and decision-making skills, such as choice of food, music, sensory reinforcers (e.g., fan, flashing lights), toys or games, social reinforcers (e.g., hugs, conversation), or video displays. Reasons for selecting the type of choices assessed in the reviewed studies included (1) availability and ease of presentation, (2) teacher nomination, (3) IEP requirements, and (4) replication of previous studies. Although these studies provided guidelines for assessing a variety of potential preferences, they did not systematically address choice in relation to more global outcomes, such as a person's lifestyle interests or preferences.

Only a handful of studies have assessed preferences in relation to everyday activities, such as fixing meals or exercising (e.g., Newton & Duda, 1993), or choice of job tasks, such as housekeeping or food service (e.g., Martin et al., 2002, 2005). Even fewer studies have looked at major lifestyle decisions, such as choosing with whom to live, moving to another community, or changing careers (e.g., Foxx, Faw, Taylor, Davis, & Fulia, 1993). Although few guidelines exist in the empirical literature for assessing lifestyle choices (Lohrmann-O'Rourke & Gomez, 2001), some programs have been developed, such as Foxx and colleagues' (1993) strategies for assessing the residential preferences of individuals with intellectual disabilities who are moving from institutions into the community, and Martin and colleagues' (2002) use of illustrations and computer-aided choice making combined with community validation of choice to decide on vocational placements (Martin, Marshall, Wray, et al., 2004).

Manner of Presenting Choices

In most of the reviewed studies, choices were assessed by placing an option on a table, wheelchair tray, or other surface in front of a participant. Teachers may also demonstrate the use of an item or activity, request a student to perform a task, or simply ask students about their preference for a particular option, with or without presenting an object representative of the option in question. Hanley and colleagues (2006) found that paired-item assessment produced the longest-lasting preference assessment results. The next section addresses how caregivers, teachers, and others may help students with disabilities learn to make choices.

TEACHING CHOICE MAKING

Studies that have investigated the development of choice-making skills stress the importance of systematically providing contingent consequences to emerging choice responses (Sigafoos & Dempsey, 1992). Sigafoos and Dempsey (1992) argued that behaviors such as approaching or reaching for a preferred item could be shaped as choice-making responses by systematically providing access to the chosen item after the response was made. For example, to teach students to make choices by manipulating electronic microswitches, Dattilo and Mirenda (1987) used computers to provide immediate access to a chosen item following a student's activation of a microswitch. The principle of providing contingent access to a preferred item or activity following a choice-making response is basic to all approaches that teach choice making. A description of some of these approaches follows.

Making Leisure Time Choices

A number of studies have used the choice-training procedure developed by Wuerch and Voeltz (1982) to teach students with intellectual disabilities to make choices related to leisure activities (e.g., Sigafoos, Roberts, Couzens, & Kerr, 1993). This procedure involves providing students with a choice of two or more previously acquired leisure activities and reinforcing them when they make a choice or prompting them when they do not. Subsequently, students are given access to the chosen activity and prompted to engage in it for increasing periods of time. "Choice charts" were used by Nietupski and colleagues (1986) to provide pictorial and written examples of leisure activities (e.g., video games, magazines, stationary bicycle) when implementing the choice-training procedure with teenagers with intellectual disabilities. Choice training resulted in increased choice of and sustained engagement in leisure activities with decreased teacher assistance for all participants. In a similar fashion, Bambara and Ager (1992) used cards that contained pictures or words that described leisure activities to help three adults with intellectual disabilities choose which activities they wished to engage in. Participants learned to use the cards to choose and schedule weekly leisure activities. Self-scheduling resulted in increased time spent engaged in chosen activities and a wider variety of activities for all participants.

Kennedy and Haring (1993) taught four students with multiple disabilities to use a microswitch communication system to request changes in leisure activities in which they were engaged with a partner. Prompting and reinforcement procedures were used to teach students to press a microswitch that activated a tape-recorded message requesting a change in activities (e.g., "Can we do something else?"). Choice-making training resulted in increases in diversity of activities chosen, time engaged in activities, and interactions with social partners.

Making Shopping Choices

As a component of a consumer education program designed to teach students with disabilities to make informed decisions when shopping, Koorland and Cooke (1990) developed a choice-making program for comparative shopping. For example, in teaching students to choose a neighborhood convenience store at which to shop, a teacher might begin by leading a class discussion on the characteristics of convenience stores that should be considered in making a choice. Based on this discussion, students develop a form to use to rate stores on identified characteristics, then shop at selected neighborhood stores and rate them. After each student picks his or her favorite store, he or she visits that store again and shops for desired items.

Making Mealtime Choices

Several studies have investigated teaching people with intellectual disabilities to exercise choice at mealtimes. Parsons and colleagues (Parsons & Reid, 1990; Parsons, McCarn, & Reid, 1993) provided adults with multiple disabilities opportunities to choose between two food or drink items throughout a meal. Participants were prompted to choose an item if they did not do so independently. Once chosen, the item was immediately provided to the participant. Findings of both studies revealed that providing access to a choice immediately following a choice response resulted in increases in choice making by all participants. Gothelf, Crimmins, Mercer, and Finocchiaro (1994) used a similar method to teach mealtime choice making to students who were deaf, blind, and had multiple disabilities. Tactile cues and physical guidance were provided to accommodate the students' sensory impairments and, upon choosing a sample of an item, students were provided with a full portion of the chosen food.

Making Lifestyle Choices

Hughes and Carter (2000) introduced a model adapted from Mithaug, Martin, and Agran's (1987) Adaptability Model to assist students in making lifestyle choices. Hughes and Carter's Choice-Making Self-Check comprises nine steps:

1. Identify my goal.
2. List my options.
3. List possible consequences of the options.
4. Choose the best option.
5. Act on the option I chose.
6. Evaluate my performance.
7. Decide if I met my goal.
8. If I didn't, go back to Step 1.
9. If I did meet my goal, remember to reward myself.

A checklist is provided, and the wording and steps are adapted to students' individual needs and skills. Students are prompted and reinforced for performing each step of the model, and attention is paid to matching choice-making responses to the student's primary communication mode and skills. Some students may learn to use the checklist independently to make various lifestyle choices such as choosing a housemate or a new hairstyle.

Faw, Davis, and Peck (1996) replicated the lifestyle choice program developed by Foxx and colleagues (1993) by teaching four adults with intellectual disabilities and mental illness to evaluate available residential options upon leaving an institution. Participants were taught to evaluate options from photographs that depicted residential characteristics. Subsequently, all participants visited the community and successfully made residential choices based on the evaluation criteria they were taught to use.

Making Employment Choices

Several educators have developed curricula for teaching students to make employment choices by sampling a variety of jobs throughout their high school years. Hutchins and Renzaglia (1990) developed a longitudinal employment-training program in which teachers evaluate students' performance on a variety of jobs over several years. Students have the opportunity to choose jobs that they would like to experience, and, based on their performance, teachers try to match students' job choices to their preferences, interests, and performance. Neubert, Danehey, and Taymans (1990) used a similar "job try-outs" program to match the employment choices of students with disabilities to job placements. Having the opportunity to sample varied jobs resulted in appropriate job matches for students that honored their vocational choices. Hagner and Salomone (1989) argued that all people base their choices for a career on their work experiences and that the opportunity to sample a variety of jobs must be provided in order for them to gather information needed to make an informed career choice.

Martin and colleagues (2002) and Martin, Valenzuela, and colleagues (2004) developed and validated an approach using illustrations or video presented in a paired-item format to assess vocational choices. Participants completed a self-determination-oriented choose, try-it, adjust, and choose again cycle until consistent preference patterns emerged.

Summary of Findings on Teaching Choice Making

Teaching choice making requires providing students with intellectual and developmental disabilities the opportunity to sample many options. For some students, choice-making responses must be shaped. In teaching choice making to students with disabilities, teachers must be careful that choice-making responses consistently are followed by access to the chosen item, activity, or event. Choice-making programs that have been investigated empirically have addressed diverse areas, such as leisure activities, lifestyle choices, and career options.

INFUSING CHOICE MAKING INTO CLASSROOM INSTRUCTION

Many researchers have emphasized the importance of learning choice-making skills in contexts that promote generalization and provide real-life opportunities to experience choices (e.g., Bambara & Ager, 1992; Dibley & Lim, 1999; Lohrmann-O'Rourke & Gomez, 2001). Shevin and Klein (1984, p. 164), in a seminal article on choice making, stressed integrating choice-making opportunities throughout the school day and listed five keys to maintaining a balance between student choice and professional responsibility:

1. Incorporating student choice as an early step in the instructional process.
2. Increasing the number of decisions the student makes related to a given activity.
3. Increasing the number of domains in which decisions are made.
4. Raising the significance in terms of risk and long-term consequences of the choices the student makes.
5. Maintaining clear communication with the student concerning areas of possible choice and the limits within which choices can be made.

Kohn (1993) suggested that school programs can provide opportunities for meaningful choices in both academic and behavioral areas. In academic areas, students can participate in choosing what, how, and why they learn. The determination of what one learns is fairly straightforward and has become a key element in promoting student involvement in educational planning and decision making (Martin, Marshall, & Maxson, 1993). Allowing a student to choose how he or she learns certainly entails more dedication and effort on the part of the teacher, but it is reasonable to provide a choice among working alone, in small groups, or as a class or to provide alternatives for where students sit while they work (Kohn, 1993).

Perhaps the most overlooked aspect of structuring choice in the classroom is getting students involved in a discussion of why they are learning. Deci and Chandler (1986) suggested that providing a rationale to learners for activities is one important way of increasing student motivation to learn and participate. Telling students that they have to learn something for their own good or other teacher-centered reasons likely will limit student self-determination. Deci and Chandler (1986) suggested that being honest and straightforward about rationales for specific learning activities moves those activities from being externally imposed to being self-regulated.

SUMMARY

Incorporating a student's preferences and choices into his or her IEP is mandated by current legislation. Historically, students with disabilities have been given limited opportunity to express preferences or exercise choices, but a growing empirical research base indicates that students with intellectual and developmental disabilities, including those with significant disabilities, can communicate their preferences and learn to make choices. The challenge for teachers and caregivers is to incorporate opportunities for these students to express their preferences and make choices throughout their daily activities (Bambara, 2004; Mithaug, 2005). Brown, Belz, Corsi, and Wenig (1993) developed a Model of Choice Diversity for embedding choice-making opportunities throughout the natural course of a student's day. The model delineated seven potential areas of choice within an activity: (1) choice of materials, (2) choice among different activities, (3) choice to refuse to participate in an activity, (4) choice of people to be included in or excluded from an activity, (5) choice of location of an activity, (6) choice of time an activity should occur, and (7) choice to end a particular activity. In planning and implementing curricula, teachers should attempt to incorporate opportunities for choice in as many of these dimensions as possible. In addition, teachers should be ready to provide instruction in choice making and expressing preferences to those students who have not yet acquired such skills. Finally, teachers should evaluate the effects on students of choice making, such as decreases in challenging behavior, increased motivation, and academic improvement.

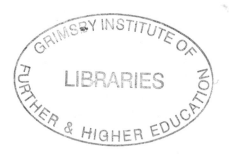

CHAPTER 3

Teaching Problem Solving and Decision Making

A student's capacity to solve problems is critical to his or her success in education and in life. This capacity has become even more important in the context of educational reform efforts. Peterson (1996) noted that an increased focus on teaching critical thinking and problem-solving skills has been central to school curriculum reform, as such skills provide the basis for all learning. Indeed, the ability to retrieve and process information and, in turn, propose a solution to a discernible problem represents a skill that greatly advances a student's competence and independence. Another critical thinking skill is the capacity to make decisions. Tymchuk (1985) noted:

> People, regardless of whether they have learning or behavior problems or are developmentally disabled, are capable of understanding consequences of their actions and can learn how to make effective decisions. Effective decision making is easily the most critical skill that anyone can learn. (p. 4)

These two skill areas—problem solving and decision making—are equally important for students to address if they are to become self-determined. Beyth-Marom, Fischhoff, Jacobs Quadrel, and Furby (1991) suggested that programs that address these skills can be classified according to (1) their focus (social or cognitive) or (2) their scope (general or specific). General social programs address interpersonal problem-solving skills, like coping strategies, assertiveness, and decision-making methods. Specific social programs focus on specific problems, such as smoking, peer and family relationships, sexuality, and physical health. Cognitive programs stress thinking skills related to the decision-making process. General cognitive programs teach decision making and problem solving among many critical thinking skills, while specific cognitive programs teach only decision making or only problem solving. This chapter will cover both social and cognitive decision-making and problem-solving strategies.

CONCEPTUALIZING PROBLEM SOLVING AND DECISION MAKING

Problem Solving

Problem solving involves using available information to identify and design solutions to problems. A "problem" is a task, activity, or situation for which a solution is not immediately identified, known, or obtainable. Solving a problem, therefore, is the process of identifying a solution that resolves the initial perplexity or difficulty. Most of the research in teaching problem solving has derived from the work of D'Zurilla (D'Zurilla, 1986; D'Zurilla & Goldfried, 1971) and Spivack, Shure, and colleagues (Shure, Spivack, & Jaeger, 1972; Spivack & Shure, 1974). D'Zurilla and Goldfried (1971) suggested a four-step training model: (1) describe the problem; (2) generate multiple response alternatives; (3) select the best solution; and (4) verify the effectiveness of the selected solution. Foxx and Faw (2000) challenged the efficacy of this cognitively based model in situations in which one must respond quickly:

> Such problems include a cashier overcharging subjects for items purchased . . . and accusations of defacing, stealing or deliberately bumping into someone. In situations such as these, the process of problem identification, goal definition, solution evaluation, evaluation of alternatives, and selection of a best solution may prove to be somewhat cumbersome and impractical. (p. 77)

Foxx and Faw (2000) suggested that an alternative is to teach students to ask a series of three questions: Who should I talk to? Where should I look for help? What should I say?. These approaches to teaching problem solving reflect different perspectives on its nature. The first views the process as primarily cognitively based, and the second as a strategy similar to self-instruction. Each has generated ideas for practice.

Decision Making

A "decision" is a process involving a broad set of skills that incorporate problem solving and choice making to select one of several already identified options. Beyth-Marom and colleagues (1991, p. 21) suggested that the decision-making process includes some basic steps:

1. Listing relevant action alternatives.
2. Identifying possible consequences of those actions.
3. Assessing the probability of each consequence occurring (if the action were undertaken).
4. Establishing the relative importance (value or utility) of each consequence.
5. Integrating these values and probabilities to identify the most attractive course of action.

These steps are similar to those identified in the problem-solving process by D'Zurilla and Goldfried except that they start by listing already identified action alternatives—that is, the decision-making process begins with the problem already solved. In addition to these core steps, there are several others that are specific to particular circumstances, including an initial step in which the individual distinguishes between different decision-making models based on circumstances. Simply put, while the core steps remain constant no matter what decisions are made, there are differences in the process based on issues of certainty/uncertainty and degree of risk.

Beyth-Marom and colleagues (1991) pointed out that uncertainty is a basic element in many decisions. Research indicates that adults and children alike tend to underestimate uncertainty in most decisions, often leading to less than optimal outcomes. There are numerous sources of uncertainty in any decision. Identifying the consequences of any given alternative is usually a best-guess situation, which may result from a lack of information about a particular option or may be a factor of the type of alternative. It is also often the case that there is uncertainty as to whether a particular alternative is actually available or will be available after a decision is made. The degree of uncertainty in each of these steps should be treated as a factor in reaching a decision, and the fact that such uncertainty typically exists should be a topic of instruction for students with disabilities.

Beyth-Marom and colleagues (1991) suggested that instruction that focuses on teaching students about uncertainty should address questions like

1. What is uncertainty?
2. What are the different kinds of uncertainty?
3. What is the relationship between uncertainty and amount of information?

Another factor that affects the decision-making process is the amount of risk involved in making a particular decision. Schloss, Alper, and Jayne (1994) detailed four levels of risk taking associated with making a choice:

1. *The alternative involves limited potential for immediate risk but little possibility of long-term harm to the individual or others.* Examples include choosing what to eat or wear. This first step also emphasizes that almost no choice is risk-free. For example, choosing to wear one's hair in a nontraditional manner may

result in others making judgments and holding expectations that are limiting or unfair.

2. *The alternative involves mild risk with minimal possibility of long-lasting harm to the individual or others.* An example is choosing to spend one's lunch money on a video game and, as a result, having to go without lunch (Schloss et al., 1994, p. 218).

3. *The alternative results in a moderate probability for long-lasting harm to the individual or others.* Examples include becoming sexually active without adequate birth control (moderate risk of becoming pregnant) and choosing to smoke cigarettes (moderate risk of cancer or other illness).

4. *The alternative involves an almost certain outcome that includes personal injury.* Schloss and colleagues (1994) identify daily use of addictive substances as an example of this level. Another example might be unprotected sexual contact with multiple partners over a long period of time (risk of HIV infection).

PROBLEM SOLVING AND STUDENTS WITH INTELLECTUAL AND DEVELOPMENTAL DISABILITIES

Like research efforts with students and individuals without disabilities, investigations of problem solving for individuals with intellectual disabilities have moved from impersonal to personal contexts. Much of this research has examined the capacity of individuals with intellectual disabilities to solve problems and has suggested that people with intellectual disabilities exhibit a largely inflexible pattern of problem-solving skills (Ellis, Woodley-Zanthos, Dulaney & Palmer, 1989; Ferretti & Butterfield, 1989; Ferretti & Cavelier, 1991; Short & Evans, 1990). This pattern "is characterized by repetition of past strategies to solve current problems without adapting to new stimuli or new task demands" (Short & Evans, 1990, p. 95). Wehmeyer and Kelchner (1994) examined the social problem-solving skills of adults with intellectual disabilities and found that this group generated fewer potential solutions to social problems and that a greater proportion of the solutions generated were irrelevant. Gumpel, Tappe, and Araki (2000) compared the social problem solving of adults with and without developmental disabilities and found that adults with developmental disabilities exhibited greater difficulty solving social problems related to employment and vocational outcomes than did nondisabled peers. In summary, educators should be aware that students with intellectual and developmental disabilities may approach problems with a limited repertoire of potential solutions and a more rigid approach to the process (e.g., relying on past strategies) and may generate more irrelevant solutions. This said, there is evidence that people with intellectual and developmental disabilities can learn more effective problem-solving skills.

Castles and Glass (1986) found that training improved social problem-solving skills of youth with mild and moderate mental retardation. Browning and Nave

(1993) used a video-based curriculum to teach social problem-solving skills to youth with mild mental retardation and learning disabilities. Bambara and Gomez (2001) taught adults with moderate to severe intellectual impairments a self-instruction process incorporating problem-solving skills. They embedded problems within the context of each person's daily routine. Participants were able to use the self-instruction sequence to solve the problem during training sequences, then generalized that experience to untrained situations. O'Reilly, Lancioni, and Kierans (2000) successfully implemented a social skills problem-solving intervention to teach leisure skills to adults with intellectual disabilities.

These findings were tempered by mixed results on the effectiveness of such programs when the outcome measure was an observed behavior. Coleman, Wheeler, and Webber (1993) found that social problem-solving training does not automatically result in students applying learned strategies to their everyday lives. Park and Gaylord-Ross (1989) found that the need to pair skills training with social problem-solving training is reciprocal. That is, skills instruction needs to accompany social problem-solving training in order for students to generalize problem-solving skills and social skills. Park and Gaylord-Ross (1989) compared social skills training without problem-solving training to a general social program that incorporated problem-solving training for youth with developmental disabilities. They found that the social problem-solving training procedure increased generalization and maintenance of the targeted social behaviors.

There are a few demonstrations of the efficacy of teaching problem-solving skills to promote educational or academic outcomes for students with intellectual or developmental disabilities. Agran, Blanchard, Hughes, and Wehmeyer (2002) taught four students with intellectual disabilities to use problem-solving skills to achieve self-set educational goals that related to increasing contributions to classroom discussions and increasing direction-following behavior. All students showed immediate and dramatic improvement in goal attainment as a function of their use of the problem-solving strategy. Similarly, O'Reilly, Lancioni, Gardiner, Tiernan, and Lacy (2002) implemented a problem-solving intervention that successfully taught students with intellectual disabilities appropriate classroom participation skills.

Finally, while there is ample research documenting the importance of social skills for positive adult outcomes for students with disabilities, little of that research has focused specifically on social problem solving. Healey and Masterpasqua (1992) examined the social problem solving of elementary school students with disabilities as a function of those students' adjustment to regular education classrooms. These researchers hypothesized that strong social problem-solving skills would be related to more positive peer relations and behavioral adjustment in the classroom. They found that this was the case and that classroom adjustment could be predicted by interpersonal cognitive problem-solving skills. Basquill, Nezu, Nezu, and Klein (2004) found that males with intellectual disabilities who were more aggressive had less effective problem-solving skills than their peers who did not engage in problem behavior, suggesting an inverse relationship between problem-solving capacity and engagement in problem behaviors.

DECISION MAKING AND STUDENTS WITH INTELLECTUAL AND DEVELOPMENTAL DISABILITIES

There has been relatively little research pertaining to the capacity of people with intellectual and developmental disabilities to make decisions. The exceptions involve research and model development by Tymchuk (Tymchuk, 1985; Tymchuk, Andron, & Rahbar, 1988) and by Hickson, Khemka, and colleagues (Hickson, Golden, Khemka, Urv, & Yamusah, 1998; Hickson & Khemka, 1999; Khemka, 2000; Khemka & Hickson, 2000; Khemka, Hickson, & Reynolds, 2005). This research and development illustrates the relevance of linking instruction in decision making to real-world issues and contexts.

Tymchuk and colleagues developed and evaluated the efficacy of interventions to teach women with intellectual disabilities parenting skills. Tymchuk and colleagues (1988) taught nine women with intellectual disabilities decision-making skills in a group setting, utilizing vignettes illustrating common child-raising situations. The participants' capacity to identify elements of the decision-making process and their use of these components to make decisions presented in the vignettes was significantly improved by the intervention. Tymchuk, Yokota, and Rahbar, (1990) examined the decision-making capacities of two groups of women, one group with intellectual disabilities, and found that the group with intellectual disabilities did not differ from the control group in the appropriateness of their decisions, but also did not utilize available information fully in coming to those decisions.

Hickson, Khemka, and colleagues conducted their research and intervention development in the context of decision making by women with intellectual disabilities at risk for domestic abuse. In preliminary research with males and females with intellectual disabilities, Hickson and colleagues (1998) found that adults with intellectual disabilities were at risk in scenarios involving potential risk due to making less vigilant decisions pertaining to interpersonal interactions (e.g., not determining well when the potential for harm or loss outweighed the possibility of gain). Khemka and Hickson (2000) also examined the decision-making performance of men and women with intellectual disabilities across three types of abusive situations: physical, sexual, and psychological/verbal. Participants were able to identify options that prevented these forms of abuse in roughly 65% of scenarios, but they were much more effective at making vigilant decisions in scenarios involving physical or sexual abuse than they were in scenarios involving psychological/verbal abuse. In summary, these studies found that adults with intellectual disabilities had some capacity to make decisions about their response to potentially abusive situations but clearly were at risk for abuse as a function of their less vigilant strategy use.

In a series of studies following these initial findings, these researchers showed that women with intellectual disabilities could learn independent decision-making skills that enabled them to be more vigilant in simulated situations of interpersonal interactions that contained elements of risk for abuse. Khemka (2000) developed a decision-making training approach that involved both cognitive and motivational components, finding that combining these aspects resulted in more positive outcomes. These women were able to acquire decision-making skills as a result of the training and performed significantly better choosing options that contained less risk. Khemka, Hickson, and Reynolds (2005) conducted a randomized-trial control-group-design study of a curriculum to teach women strategies to make more effective decisions and found that this process was very effective, enabling women with intellectual disabilities to acquire and use decision-making strategies that minimized their risk for potential abuse.

Both these lines of research suggest that, not surprisingly, people with intellectual disabilities who are not provided explicit instruction on decision-making skills are not as capable of making effective decisions and, in high-risk situations (such as those involving abuse) or in situations where decisions may have considerable consequences (such as parenting), are at risk for negative outcomes. It should be emphasized, however, that even in high-risk situations, which tend to be where research has been conducted, people with intellectual disabilities have been shown to have some capacity, a finding often ignored. Attention has been directed to health-care-related decisions by people with impaired capacity to make decisions, and research has begun to confirm that people with intellectual disabilities have more capacity to understand treatment options and identify appropriate courses of action pertaining to health care than previously assumed (Cea & Fisher, 2003).

Both lines of research also show that, given explicit instruction, people with intellectual disabilities can acquire the decision-making skills that enable them to perform much more effectively, even in these high-risk situations. Two recent studies on the ability of people with intellectual disabilities to make financial decisions further illustrate the growing consensus that people with intellectual disabilities have the capacity to become effective decision makers. Suto, Clare, Holland, and Watson (2005a, 2005b) examined the financial decision-making abilities of people with intellectual disabilities and nondisabled peers. These researchers found that IQ level was only partially related to a person's capacity to make financial decisions and that while the decision-making abilities of study participants with intellectual disabilities were generally weaker than those of their nondisabled peers, these differences were not dramatic.

There is, unfortunately, no research examining school-based interventions to promote the decision-making skills of students with intellectual disabilities, and while there are several interventions supported by evidence to increase decision-making skills of individuals with intellectual and developmental disabilities, they have not been evaluated in the context of educational settings. There are, however, models evaluated with other populations of students with disabilities that hypothetically would have utility with students with intellectual and developmental disabilities. Both models evaluated with adults with intellectual disabilities and with students with disabilities are discussed in the following section.

PROMOTING PROBLEM-SOLVING AND DECISION-MAKING SKILLS

Returning to the classification of the types of decision-making training approaches and strategies suggested by Beyth-Marom and colleagues (1991), this section will describe specific instructional programs and strategies that can be employed to promote student problem-solving and decision-making skills.

General Social Approaches and Strategies

General social approaches and strategies teach a wide number of interpersonal problem-solving skills, like coping strategies, assertiveness, and decision-making methods. The most common of these strategies are assertiveness-training programs and social skills–training programs. Assertiveness-training strategies consist of a number of multicomponent packages built upon behavioral rehearsal and including the basic elements of modeling, coaching, feedback, and homework assignments to teach assertive behavior. Social skills–training programs incorporate instructional elements that are also involved in the assertiveness-training process, like role playing, modeling, and rehearsal, but typically share fewer components than do different assertiveness-training programs. Social skills–training programs are often linked as much by their content (e.g., teaching social skills) as their approach. Assertiveness and effective communication skills are covered in Chapter 5.

Benjamin (1996a, 1996b) developed two general social programs that address a wide range of social and problem-solving skills at school and at work. Benjamin introduced a problem-solving plan designed to get students thinking about problems they encounter. Students are taught the following four steps (Benjamin, 1996a, p. iv):

1. *Understand*: Ask yourself, "What is the problem? What do I need to find out?"
2. *Plan and solve*: Ask yourself, "What do I already know? How will I solve this problem?" Then use problem-solving skills to help you carry out your plan.
3. *Check*: Look at what happened. Ask yourself, "Have I solved the problem? Does my plan make sense?" If there's still a problem, look over your plan. Change your plan. Try another problem-solving skill to solve the problem.
4. *Review*: Look at what you did to solve the problem. Ask yourself, "What have I learned? How can I use my plan to solve problems like this in the future?"

Areas of instruction in which this plan is applied are listed in Table 3.1. As this table shows, the skills addressed involve a wide range of social and self-advocacy

TABLE 3.1. Problem-Solving Areas in the School Environment

Unit	Instructional area
Unit 1: Preparing for School	Planning your day. Getting dressed. Morning chores. Getting to school.
Unit 2: Managing in School	Being on time. Following your schedule. Finishing your schoolwork. Taking notes. Doing homework. Studying. Class time and personal time.
Unit 3: Communication Skills	Talking with a teacher. Talking with a friend. Listening. Asking questions. Oral reports.
Unit 4: Making Judgments and Decisions	Peer pressure. Problems with students. Problems in school. Changes at school. Setting goals. School and work. Planning what schoolwork to do first.
Unit 5: Managing Money	Budgeting. Paying. Saving.

Note. From Wehmeyer, Agran, and Hughes (1998). Copyright 1998 by Michael Wehmeyer, Martin Agran, and Carolyn Hughes. Reprinted by permission.

skills, including goal setting, money management, effective communication, and planning. Benjamin (1996b) has also applied the same problem-solving plan to social skills, vocational skills, and self-advocacy skills training in the work environment, as seen in Table 3.2.

Specific Social Approaches and Strategies

Unlike general social skills approaches and strategies, which are broadly focused, specific social approaches and strategies focus on specific problems encountered by youth, such as smoking, peer and family relationships, sexuality, or physical health. Problem-solving and decision-making skills instruction occurs only as a component of addressing the specific social problem. There are numerous examples of specific social approaches and strategies used with individuals with disabilities to address problems like anger control or community living.

TABLE 3.2. Problem-Solving Areas in the Work Environment

Unit	Instructional area
Unit 1: Preparing for Work	Getting ready. Getting dressed. Getting to work.
Unit 2: Managing Time	Being on time. Your workday. Organizing work time. Work time and personal life.
Unit 3: Managing Job Duties	Completing forms. Job duties. Planning which job to do first. Completing jobs on time. Dressing for work. Finding information.
Unit 4: Communication Skills	Talking with a boss. Talking with coworkers. Talking with customers. Listening. Asking questions.
Unit 5: Making Judgments and Decisions	Peer pressure. Problems on the job. Personal issues. Change at work.
Unit 6: Managing Money	Reading a pay stub. Payday. Budgeting.

Note. From Wehmeyer, Agran, and Hughes (1998). Copyright 1998 by Michael Wehmeyer, Martin Agran, and Carolyn Hughes. Reprinted by permission.

Foxx and Bittle (1989) developed a curriculum called Thinking It Through for use with students with intellectual and developmental disabilities that teaches a problem-solving strategy for community living. The curriculum focuses on several areas that the authors identify as important to successful community adjustment, including (1) emergencies and injuries, (2) safety, (3) authority figures, (4) peer issues, (5) community resources, and (6) stating one's rights. The program "is designed to teach a problem-solving strategy by presenting trainees with commonly experienced problems and by guiding them to consider a sequence of problem-solving questions in formulating their solutions" (Foxx & Bittle, 1989, p. 4).

Instead of containing instructional activities focused on teaching students a specific cognitive process, Thinking It Through teaches students to ask a series of questions in order to formulate solutions to specific problems. There are four problem situations in each of the six areas mentioned above. The questions are listed below, and one problem situation from each area is listed in Table 3.3:

1. When will the problem be solved?
2. Where would you or a friend look for help?
3. Whom would you or your friend talk to?
4. What would you or your friend say?

Training involves the use of cue cards with one problem situation per card and is configured in a manner similar to direct instruction. The facilitator works with three participants, who each select cue cards and, based on the community-living-related problem, are asked to provide a solution. Through practice and self-monitoring for appropriate solutions, individuals build a repertoire of solutions to community-living-based problems.

Tymchuk (1985) developed an instructional process to teach decision making to persons with developmental disabilities based primarily on research in child development. Tymchuk's process identified 11 steps to effective decision making, listed in Table 3.4. Tymchuk organizes lessons around each of the steps in the process. In teaching the decision that needs to be made (Step 1), the person is presented with multiple scenarios in which a decision must be made, all of which are grounded in real-world situations (e.g., a friend asks you to smoke, someone teases you). Participants learn to brainstorm potential decisions (Step 3) and to identify

TABLE 3.3. Sample Problem Situations from Thinking It Through

General category	Sample problem situation
Emergencies and injuries	You feel very dizzy. What should you do?
Safety	You are walking outside and get caught in a thunderstorm. Your friend says, "Let's get under a tree." What should you do?
Authority figures	You just broke your supervisor's favorite mug. He is going to be angry. What should you do?
Peer issues	Whenever you go out with your friend, he burps loudly and then laughs. You are really getting embarrassed. What should you do?
Community resources	A child walks up to you at the fair and says she is lost. What should you do?
Stating one's rights	You have a friend who keeps asking you to go out on a date. You don't want to go. What should you do?

Note. From Wehmeyer, Agran, and Hughes (1998). Copyright 1998 by Michael Wehmeyer, Martin Agran, and Carolyn Hughes. Reprinted by permission.

TABLE 3.4. Steps to Effective Decision Making

Step	Action
1	Identify the decision to be made.
2	Identify who should be involved in making this decision.
3	Identify alternative decisions.
4	Identify the chain of events.
5	Identify if/then statements.
6	Identify the immediate consequences.
7	Identify the ongoing consequences.
8	Identify the long-term consequences.
9	Make a decision.
10	Evaluate whether the decision went the way you predicted.
11	Change the decision, if necessary.

Note. From Wehmeyer, Agran, and Hughes (1998). Copyright 1998 by Michael Wehmeyer, Martin Agran, and Carolyn Hughes. Reprinted by permission.

consequences associated with each decision. These consequences are both positive and negative and include immediate (Step 6), ongoing (Step 7), and long-term (Step 8) consequences. Participants are taught to consider psychological, academic, vocational, leisure, family, health, financial, and social benefits associated with the consequences. Participants also learn to consider negative consequences that involve risks in these same areas.

Bullock and Mahon (1992) developed an approach for teaching students with disabilities a decision-making process specific to leisure decisions. They began instruction with a leisure awareness–training program in which students with disabilities were introduced to five components important to leisure awareness.

1. Concepts of leisure
2. Self-awareness in leisure
3. Knowledge of leisure opportunities
4. Leisure resources
5. Leisure barriers

After students completed the leisure awareness–training module, they were taught the Decision Making in Leisure (DML) model, composed of four steps.

1. Identify a desired leisure experience.
2. Consider alternatives that satisfy the experience desired.
3. Describe the consequences for each alternative, including the amount of enjoyment, whether a partner is required, the cost, where the activity takes place, and the equipment needed.
4. Choose an alternative that satisfies the desired experience.

Instruction using the DML model involves five instructional steps.

1. *Introduce the four-step model*: Steps are introduced using both oral and pictorial presentation of each step.
2. *Teach child to use four steps to make a decision:* Students are taught to use a schematic representation of the model each time they are asked to make a decision.
3. *Teacher offers assistance when necessary*: The teacher or facilitator allows the student to work through the decision-making process but provides verbal cues to support him or her as necessary.
4. *Teacher provides verbal praise as student proceeds through decision.*
5. *Remove schematic of DML model.*

Using the DML model, Bullock and Mahon (1992) taught students with intellectual disabilities to make decisions independently about their leisure activities in classroom settings. They suggested, however, that the teaching approach could be implemented in a physical education setting or in students' homes.

General Cognitive Approaches and Strategies

Social problem-solving and decision-making approaches and strategies teach problem solving and decision making as one aspect of teaching general or specific social skills. Cognitive problem-solving and decision-making approaches and strategies focus exclusively on teaching critical thinking skills, with problem solving or decision making as one of many critical thinking skills or as the sole critical thinking skill. In reality, there is considerable overlap between cognitive and social approaches, and in many cases the assignment of a particular strategy to one or the other is somewhat arbitrary. The primary difference is one of emphasis—social skills training versus critical thinking skills training. General cognitive approaches and strategies teach problem solving and decision making as two of many critical thinking skills. One empirically validated general cognitive approach that has been validated for use with students with intellectual and developmental disabilities involves the use of the Self-Determined Learning Model of Instruction (Wehmeyer, Palmer, Agran, Mithaug, & Martin, 2000), covered in Chapter 9.

Another example of a general cognitive approach is the IDEAL Problem Solver (Bransford & Stein, 1993), a program that teaches individuals critical thinking, memory, and problem-solving skills. In this particular approach, problem-solving skills take center stage. Through the program, students learn a five-step problem-solving strategy to approach any problem. The acronym for the strategy is IDEAL, and the steps involve teaching students to:

- I = Identify problems and opportunities.
- D = Define goals.
- E = Explore possible strategies.

- A = Anticipate outcomes and act.
- L = Look back and learn.

What characterizes the IDEAL Problem Solver approach as a cognitive program is its focus on coupling other thinking skills with the IDEAL problem-solving
strategy. In the course of completing the program, participants work on strategies
that target several critical thinking skills, like memory. Participants learn categori-
zation strategies (grouping like items in order to remember them) and visualiza-
tion techniques, like the method of loci, where items to be remembered are visualized in a familiar location, or interactive imagery strategies, where items to be
remembered are paired and visualized in a manner that will be easy to recall (e.g., a
dog talking on the telephone). The program then focuses on critical thinking skills,
like using basic comprehension strategies. Bransford and Stein (1993) employed a
wide range of instructional strategies to teach these thinking skills, including case-
based instruction (organizing instruction around a situation the student is likely to
encounter), project-based instruction (organizing instruction around a student project), debates, simulations, cooperative learning, and student-directed learning
strategies.

Specific Cognitive Approaches and Strategies

Instructional approaches and strategies classified under this final category are cognitive programs that teach only (or, in reality, primarily) problem-solving or
decision-making strategies. Quite a few of these programs have evolved from the
work of D'Zurilla (1986) and Spivack and Shure (1974) discussed previously. For
example, Elias, Branden-Muller, and Sayette (1991) summarized the theoretical
approach adopted by D'Zurilla as it applied in educational settings. D'Zurilla's
problem-solving model involved five specific stages: (1) problem orientation, (2)
problem definition and formulation, (3) generation of alternative solutions, (4)
decision making, and (5) solution implementation.

According to Elias and colleagues (1991, p. 168) the problem orientation stage
has four functions:

1. To increase awareness of problems and to introduce the idea of problem
   solving.
2. To encourage positive expectations for problem solving and divert attention
   from negative or preoccupying thoughts.
3. To encourage persistence against emotional stress and difficult situations.
4. To facilitate a positive emotional state.

Several cognitive variables are targeted within the first phase. First, instruction
focuses on problem perception, or the recognition and labeling of problems. Second, instruction focuses on problem attribution skills (e.g., problems attributed to
internal or external factors) and problem appraisal skills (the individual's judg-

ment as to the importance of the problem). Participants also learn how to estimate the time they will need to solve a problem during this phase.

In the second phase, problem definition and formulation, participants learn to gather as much information about the problem as possible, set problem-solving goals, and reexamine the importance of the problem's resolution to their well-being. In phase three, individuals learn to generate alternative solutions to the problem. The generation of alternatives is a step that is often problematic for students with disabilities. As previously mentioned, students with mental retardation and learning disabilities often generate fewer appropriate alternatives than same-age peers without disabilities. Many students with disabilities tend to perseverate on alternatives that are either ineffective or share a common theme or characteristic. So, for example, students with emotional or behavioral disorders may generate multiple alternatives, all involving aggressive responses. Most people derive options based on a combination of learning and experience. Students with disabilities too often do not have the experience base from which to draw when generating alternatives, and instruction in this area may be as simple as expanding a student's experiences in areas of importance, like work or leisure.

The emergence of the ability to generate alternative solutions typically follows a specific sequence (Beyth-Marom et al., 1991). The first stage is the generation of a single alternative. Students who are not able to do so should be provided instructional opportunities that enable them to generate at least one alternative for a problem relevant to their lives. At the next stage, students learn to generate a small list of alternative solutions. Again, this may be primarily a rote exercise, learning about and memorizing several alternatives to common problems. At the next stage, students learn how to brainstorm alternatives. The final stages involve the generation of alternative solutions by classification and criteria standards (e.g., actually inventing alternatives based on characteristics of the problem situation and past experiences).

The fourth stage of the D'Zurilla problem-solving model involves decision making. Specifically, participants are taught to consider the value and likelihood of the anticipated consequences, decide whether the alternatives are feasible and acceptable, and examine the costs and benefits of the alternatives. The final stage, solution implementation and verification, incorporates several cognitive-behavioral features (as opposed to strictly cognitive features), including self-monitoring, self-evaluation, and self-reinforcement, all of which are considered in greater detail in other chapters in this text.

The approach developed and validated by Khemka and colleagues (Khemka, 2000; Khemka & Hickson, 2000; Khemka et al., 2005) falls into the category of a specific cognitive approach, although the focus on decision making is included within the context of goal setting and increasing knowledge about abuse and neglect. Their curriculum, titled an Effective Strategy-based Curriculum for Abuse Prevention and Empowerment (ESCAPE), focuses on teaching women with intellectual disabilities to make decisions in the context of interpersonal situations that pose some risk for abuse. A subsequent version, ESCAPE-DD, was developed for use with males as well as females. Within the ESCAPE process, the decision-making strategy instruction is preceded by lessons on abuse concepts to provide participants with knowledge about healthy and abusive relationships and types of abuse. The process contains both a cognitive component and an emotional/motivational component.

Instruction on decision making begins with teaching participants four steps in critical thinking pertaining to making a decision. These steps are:

1. Deciding if there is a problem and how you feel.
2. Thinking about all the choices you have.
3. Knowing what will happen with each choice and deciding if the choice meets your goals.
4. Deciding which choice is best for you and making a decision.

These cognitive steps are taught in the context of vignettes accompanied by visuals that illustrate scenarios in which a protagonist is at risk for abuse. Through scripted discussion points and brainstorming activities, participants decide if the scenario depicts a problem, talk about how they feel about the problem, and consider options the protagonist might have in the situation. The instructor repeats this process in a series of lessons that go from guided practice to collaborative group practice to participant-guided practice to independent performance.

A current application of the ESCAPE curriculum being pursued by Hickson, Khemka, and colleagues is the use of the curriculum with people with Williams syndrome, who, because of characteristics associated with their condition, including an outgoing and trusting nature, may be particularly at risk for abuse.

SUMMARY

Although the cognitive and metacognitive demands of the problem-solving and decision-making process have resulted in a generally held assumption that many individuals with intellectual and developmental disabilities cannot learn to make decisions or solve problems, research and model development have shown otherwise. It is clear, however, that unless they receive explicit instruction in these critical thinking skill areas, students with disabilities will not be able to meet the problem-solving or decision-making demands in their educational or other environments. There are numerous validated approaches and strategies to teaching problem solving and decision making, within both social and cognitive frameworks and either embedded with other social or critical thinking skills or taught individually. In all contexts, though, these are skills that should be taught addressing contexts and situations that are both meaningful and anchored in reality so as to encourage generalization.

CHAPTER 4

Teaching Goal Setting and Attainment

In Chapter 1, we suggested that two of the defining features of self-determined behavior are its volitional nature and its intentionality. At the heart of intentional behavior—and self-determined behavior—is goal-oriented action. A goal is an outcome that is the target of one's actions. Goal-setting and attainment skills enable students to determine and set a goal, to develop a plan to achieve that goal, and to monitor and adjust that goal or plan accordingly. In Chapter 9, we discuss an instructional model that teaches students a self-regulated problem-solving process to enable them to set and achieve goals. In this chapter, we discuss goal setting and attainment more specifically.

CONCEPTUALIZING GOAL SETTING AND ATTAINMENT

A variety of terms have been used to refer to the process of setting a goal (e.g., self-selection of performance standards, goal attainment, self-determination of contingencies), and varied interpretations of the purpose of goals in governing human behavior and the process of goal setting, based upon differing theoretical perspectives, have been offered.

Goal Setting and Self-Regulation Theory

Goal setting is a central feature of self-regulation theory (Zimmerman, Bandura, & Martinez-Pons, 1992). Self-regulation relies on self-monitoring, and goals determine the standards by which one compares one's current performance to one's desired outcome or goal state (Zimmerman, Bonner, & Kovach, 1996). Goal-setting theory is built on the underlying assumption that goals are regulators of human action. Research in goal orientation theory (Ames, 1992; Dweck, 1986) has focused on differences in achievement as a function of the type of the goal set, whether task or performance. Examining the impact of goals on work productivity within a self-regulation framework, Locke and Latham (2002) documented the mechanisms by which goals operate, examined moderators of goal effectiveness, and explored the relationship between goals and satisfaction. Although none of this research has been specifically applied to students with intellectual and developmental disabilities, it is important to summarize its findings (Locke & Latham, 1990, 2002).

1. People perform more effectively under goal conditions than under nongoal conditions. The research suggests that setting goals regulates effort expended and persistence.
2. Goal specificity or clarity affects performance. Clearly articulated, measurable goals enhance performance more than nonquantified or nonspecific goals.
3. Goal difficulty is related to performance. Harder (though attainable) goals lead to greater effort, persistence, and enhanced performance compared to easier goals.
4. Goals affect performance because they "direct attention and effort toward goal-relevant activities and away from goal-irrelevant activities" (Locke & Latham, 2002, p. 706).
5. Goal performance outcomes are strongest when people are committed to their goals. Goal commitment is a function of the importance of the goal to the person and his or her belief that he or she can attain the goal.
6. Goal attainment is linked to effective feedback on goal progress.

Johnson and Graham (1990) identified other properties that differentiate among goals and affect their acquisition. In addition to specificity and difficulty, these authors identified proximity as a factor in goal attainment. Goals can be "proximal" (near in time) or "distal" (far off in time). Proximal goals are associated with higher goal performance than distal goals (Johnson & Graham, 1990). Johnson and Graham also identified a factor that has some mixed findings in the literature: the impact of self-set versus other-set goals on performance. Locke and Latham (2002) found that workers performed equally well under self-set and other-set goal conditions. Upon further exploration, they determined that this was only the case when the other-set goal was delivered with a clear explanation as to why that performance target was set; otherwise, the self-set goal was related to higher performance. Given the importance of student involvement in educational planning and decision making in special education (discussed in detail in Chapter 11), this factor warrants consideration, and while the findings are not unequivocal, there is evidence in the special education literature that students perform better when they are involved in goal setting (Johnson & Graham, 1990).

Goal Setting and Behavioral Theory

A behavioral explanation of the goal-setting process emphasizes that people must be aware of both the consequences of their actions and the contingencies operating in their environments (Miller & Kelly, 1994). In addition, to gain access to the delayed reinforcement of a long-term goal (e.g., graduating from high school in 4 years), a student must relinquish continual access to competing, powerful, immediate consequences (e.g., going skiing for the weekend rather than studying for finals). Over time, acting to obtain immediate reinforcement could result in consequences that would preclude access to long-term goals.

Individuals face a dilemma when setting and pursuing a goal because they must choose between two or more actions that have different consequences, both immediate and delayed (Hughes & Lloyd, 1993). For example, a student may have a goal of saving money to purchase a car but may be tempted to use her weekly paycheck immediately to buy CDs. This situation presents a conflict to the student because the effects of the two responses occur at different times. In contrast, if opportunities (e.g., a limitless supply of funds) to buy a car or purchase CDs occurred at the same time, there would be no dilemma. The student would simply choose a purchase based upon personal preference. The dilemma occurs because a preferred activity for an individual (such as spending one's money) provides immediate reinforcement, whereas the effect of not saving funds (e.g., not enough money is accumulated to buy a car) is experienced only after a delay (Bandura, 1969). The difference between immediate and delayed consequences makes goal setting and attainment difficult for many people.

A potential solution to the dilemma of delayed reinforcers, according to behaviorists, is to make certain people are aware of the contingencies in effect in their environment (Baer, 1984). This learning may be facilitated by making the consequences of actions more salient (Hughes & Lloyd, 1993). For example, to prompt studying, students could be informed that the result of continued poor grades will be academic probation and eventual dismissal from school.

A second solution to the dilemma is to have a student sign a behavioral contract when the perceived value of the delayed outcome of the goal is high. For example, Rachlin (1978) suggested that a student sign a written contract stating a contingency such as loss of privileges or money for not studying. The contract should be signed when the student's perceived value of studying is high (e.g., when the student's goal of obtaining a scholarship is contingent on maintaining good grades), and it decreases the student's potential choices due to the possible loss of privileges during those times when the value of studying may wane (e.g., when there are competing reinforcers).

A third solution is teaching students to use self-management techniques to delay their reinforcers when pursuing a goal (Hughes & Lloyd, 1993). Through the use of direct instructional principles such as prompting, modeling, practice, and corrective feedback, people have been taught to modify their behavior by observing instances of their failure to delay reinforcers (e.g., eating three scoops of ice cream when attempting to lose weight) and the environmental events affecting their behavior (e.g., overeating as a result of a stressful day at work). Bandura (1969) emphasized that "the goals that individuals choose for themselves must be specified sufficiently . . . to provide adequate guidance for the actions that must be taken daily to attain desired outcomes" (p. 255). The use of a recording device (e.g., daily log) may help make environmental events and their consequences more salient to the individual. In addition, a student's actions may be brought under the control of long-term consequences by employing techniques such as:

1. Commitment strategies (e.g., arranging to have a wake-up call in order to arrive at an appointment on time)
2. Rules and verbal behavior (e.g., raising one's hand before speaking in class to avoid loss of privileges)
3. Stimulus control (e.g., eating only when sitting at a table to avoid snacking between meals)
4. Public announcement of goals (e.g., stating publicly the intention to quit smoking)

GOAL SETTING AND STUDENTS WITH INTELLECTUAL AND DEVELOPMENTAL DISABILITIES

Goal setting has been linked to successful outcomes for students with disabilities, particularly adult and academic outcomes for students with learning disabilities (Graham, MacArthur, & Schwartz, 1995; Graham, MacArthur, Schwartz, & Page-Voth, 1992; Lenz, Ehren, & Smiley, 1991; Johnson, Graham, & Harris, 1997; Page-Voth & Graham, 1999; Raskind, Goldberg, Higgins, & Herman, 2002; Troia & Graham, 2002), though some studies have shown the efficacy of goal setting for students with emotional and behavioral disorders as well (Ruth, 1996; Zaragoza, Vaughn, & McIntosh, 1991).

In most of these studies, goal setting was implemented along with other learning strategies as a part of a multicomponent intervention to affect content attainment and academic performance. The literature specifically pertaining to goal setting and students with intellectual disabilities is similar in some ways and different in others. Copeland and Hughes (2002) reviewed empirical investigations of the effects of goal setting on task performance of persons with intellectual disabilities and identified 17 articles with either group-experimental-design or single-subject–design studies, many of which employed goal setting as a part of a multicomponent intervention. In 15 of these 17 research reports, task performance either increased or improved following goal-setting training (Copeland & Hughes, 2002, p. 49).

To some degree, that is where similarities between knowledge about the impact of goal setting on outcomes for students with intellectual disabilities and knowledge about the impact of goal setting on outcomes for students with other disabilities ends. Despite the modest but sufficient number of studies reporting the positive impact of goal setting on task performance for persons with intellectual disabilities, Copeland and Hughes (2002) found that the outcomes targeted by goal setting as an intervention were surprisingly limited. Sixty-five percent looked at the impact of goal setting on rate and accuracy of sorting and assembly tasks. These were mainly older studies focused on improving the performance of people with intellectual disabilities on tasks common in sheltered employment, an outcome that is not currently desired. In fact, only two studies examined the impact of goals on academic tasks for this population. Gardner and Gardner (1978) incorporated goal setting as an instructional strategy to improve performance on spelling and vocabulary tests and found that students provided direct instruction on goal setting scored significantly higher on both spelling and vocabulary posttests. Warner and DeJung (1971) examined goal and no-goal groups' performance on spelling tasks and found that the goal-setting group performed significantly better on a spelling posttest, although there were no effects of hard versus easy goals.

The fact that there have been so few empirical evaluations of the impact of goal setting on academic achievement or, for that matter, on any outcome for students with intellectual disabilities is discouraging, but the overwhelmingly positive impact of goal setting on task attainment in the extant studies gives cause for optimism. Further, in research reported more extensively in Chapter 9, Wehmeyer, Palmer, Agran, Mithaug, and Martin (2000) incorporated goal-setting instruction into a multicomponent model of teaching to promote self-directed learning and self-regulated problem solving and provided evidence that students with intellectual disabilities can set and achieve educationally valid goals. Wehmeyer and colleagues (2000) examined the impact of teaching students a self-regulated problem-solving process (which began with students identifying and setting a goal and included the development of an action plan to meet that goal and a process for monitoring and evaluating progress toward the goal) on the goal attainment of 40 students with intellectual disabilities, learning disabilities, or emotional and behavioral disorders. These 40 students set 43 goals, 10 of which focused on acquiring or modifying social skills or knowledge, 13 on behavioral issues (compliance with school procedures, controlling behavior in specific circumstances, learning more adaptive behavior), and 20 on academic needs. Overall, more than 80% of students involved in the study made at least some progress toward their goal receiving instruction using the model, and 55% achieved or exceeded their goal.

Agran, Blanchard, and Wehmeyer (2000) examined the goal attainment of 19 middle school and high school students with disabilities—13 students with an intellectual disability, 3 students with a learning disability, and the other 3 with multiple disabilities—who received instruction using the model. Sixty-eight percent of the 19 goals set were attained at a satisfactory level or higher, and only 10% of the students ($n = 2$) made no progress on their goal. Finally, Palmer, Wehmeyer, Gibson, and Agran (2004) examined the impact of instruction using the model with 22 middle school students with intellectual disabilities who, consistent with previous research, showed high rates of goal attainment.

In summary, it is evident that students with intellectual and developmental disabilities can participate in the goal-setting process and in doing so achieve both academic and functional skills benefit. There is, however, a need for research to examine in greater detail what aspects of goals contribute to greater goal attainment for this population.

TEACHING GOAL-SETTING AND ATTAINMENT SKILLS

Teaching students to set goals involves instruction on a series of steps that move them from goal identification to goal articulation. There are obviously many domains in which goals can be written, but to illustrate the process of teaching students to set and attain a goal, we will focus only on learning goals.

Teaching Goal-Setting Skills

Step 1: Identify the Goal

The first step in setting a goal is to identify the goal or target. Have students think about what they want or need to learn. This may be as straightforward as identifying the student performance standards associated with a given content area, or students may need to consider their present knowledge of content information or skills to identify the next step in the learning process.

Step 2: Write the Goal

Having the student write (or dictate) a goal serves a number of purposes, including making it more real to the student, ensuring that the goal will not be forgotten, and providing a starting point for refining the goal. To begin, have the student write what he or she sees as the goal. Then work with the student to expand or revise the goal to ensure the following characteristics or features:

• *Is the goal so clear and specific that students know immediately whether or not they have met it?* Sands and Doll (2005) noted that students may have a tendency to express goals in vague or broad terms. As a starting point, students need to refine their goal to be sure that behaviors and outcomes are clear and stated precisely. For performance goals, the outcome must be clearly and specifically described. For process goals, the actions or processes to be implemented must, likewise, be clear and specific. Goal specificity can be linked to goal measurability, as discussed subsequently.

Kish (1991) noted a number of potential barriers to setting clear and specific goals.

1. *Lack of knowledge and information*: Some adolescents cannot set goals because they lack information or knowledge. Providing necessary information is an important step in the goal-setting process because it may help students develop a new perspective on their problems.
2. *Lack of skills*: A lack of skills may prevent students from setting and attaining goals. Teachers may need to help students develop specific skills such as assertiveness, problem solving, self-management, communication, and decision making in order to proceed with the goal-setting process.
3. *Fear of risk taking*: Fear of taking risks may interfere with goal setting. Teachers may need to help students overcome their fear of risk taking through strategies such as role play.
4. *Lack of social supports*: Students with disabilities too often have few supportive relationships. Helping them develop support networks may facilitate goal attainment.

A study by Balcazar, Keys, and Garate-Serafini (1995) with six students with learning disabilities highlights the effectiveness of instruction in skills related to the four barriers listed above. These students with disabilities received support to facilitate goal setting and completion for transition-related goals. The exercise of setting goals was enhanced by teaching related social activities that involved finding assistance to aid in goal completion, sometimes in situations where students did not have contact with family or friends. The goals were met and social competencies generalized to other situations beyond the specific goals that were attained, supporting the effectiveness of instruction in goal-related strategies.

• *Is there a time established for the accomplishment of the goal?* Goals only regulate behavior when they cause us to act, and setting specific deadlines by which to achieve a goal or steps in the goal is one way to regulate our action. Research discussed previously (Johnson & Graham, 1990) showed that shorter-duration goals were more likely to be linked to positive performance. Further, students with intellectual disabilities may have difficulty conceptualizing time and may not understand the time frame within which longer-term goals should be achieved. It is important to assist students to set timelines that are more immediate, which dictates that the action or target of the goal be achievable in a relatively short time.

In some cases, it may be most effective to have the goal delineate a starting date as well as a completion date. A start time, date, or event provides impetus to begin working toward a goal. The start date should be in the near future. If it is in the too distant future, the goal may be forgotten or may no longer be appropriate when the time comes to start working on it. Starting and completion dates are also helpful in calculating total time for goal attainment.

- *Is the goal measurable?* Clarity and specificity are important so that students know when they've achieved a goal, and such progress should be measurable. Goals should be defined in terms of observable or measurable outcomes. Encourage the use of specific measures (e.g., frequency or percentage correct, hours of effort, etc.) so that it will be easy to determine when the goal is met.

- *Can the goal be broken into component steps or objectives?* Objectives are the actions or steps needed to achieve a goal. The process of laying out objectives may also be helpful in evaluating the appropriateness of a goal. If there are too many objectives, maybe the goal is too complex and needs to be broken into several smaller goals. A well-defined goal will have clear objectives that are easily measurable.

- *Is the goal written to be positive and future-oriented?* Goals should be written in a positive manner. The goal should project something that is increased, gained, or added rather than something that is restricted, taken away, or reduced. The goal should result in something good, such as better health, greater professional expertise, or a more organized office that can be attained in the future.

- *Is the goal attainable?* This question may sound redundant to previous considerations, but it is worth considering on its own merit. Certainly aspects such as completion time and goal measurability will come into play with regard to goal attainment, but there are other factors that impact attainability as well. For example, is the goal something that the student has control over and can modify, change, or otherwise ensure progress? Another factor might be that the goal is too advanced. Again, research shows that harder (though still attainable) goals lead to greater effort, persistence, and enhanced performance when compared to easier goals, but goals that are too hard or too far away from attainment decrease motivation and persistence.

Teaching Goal Attainment

Once the student has set a goal that takes into account the conditions above he or she must then focus on attaining that goal. This process involves several more steps.

Step 3: Create an Action Plan

An action plan describes the strategies students will implement to achieve the goal they have set and establishes how they will monitor progress. A student should consider some of the following issues when creating an action plan:

- *What strategies or actions will be needed to achieve the goal?* Teachers should help students identify instructional and other strategies (in the case of learning goals) or actions that will help them close the gap between their current performance or mastery and their goal performance level. Sometimes those actions involve acquisition of new knowledge and skills, and in many cases students don't know all the strategies they can use to acquire that knowledge and skills. Teachers can provide that information.

• *What resources will be needed to implement the action plan?* Resources can be broadly cast to include needed materials, transportation, and adult or peer assistance. The action plan should include information on resources needed and how those resources will be obtained.

• *What schedule will be needed to implement the strategies or actions?* Students need to determine how often and when they are going to work on the activities leading to the goal. Teaching students self-scheduling procedures can be valuable in this context.

• *What process will be used to measure time spent implementing the action plan?* Students will need to track how often they work on their action plan so that, when they evaluate their progress toward the goal, they can decide if their commitment to the action plan has been sufficient.

• *What self-monitoring strategy will be implemented to monitor progress?* Every action plan should include a specific self-monitoring strategy that will enable students to collect data with regard to their goal attainment progress. Because self-monitoring is discussed in detail in Chapter 7, we will not go into detail here, other than to note that it is important to establish baseline levels of performance using these self-monitoring strategies, with which students can compare future performance.

• *What other sources of feedback can provide information about progress?* In addition to the data generated through self-monitoring, there may be other sources of data or feedback that students can tap into that will make their self-evaluation more effective.

• *What schedule will be needed to track progress toward the goal?* Just as student engagement in activities specified in the action plan should be scheduled, so should intervals at which data will be collected. In general, more frequent data collection is preferable. Teachers can work with students to teach them how to record the data they are gathering in ways that will assist in evaluating their progress.

Step 4: Evaluate Progress and Adjust Plan or Goal

In evaluating their progress toward their goal, students should be taught to use data collected through the self-monitoring process and through other means to determine answers to the following questions:

• *Is my progress adequate?* All of the self-evaluation processes involve comparing current status to goal status. Students should use data collected to determine if they have reached their goal. If not, they need to determine if they have made progress from baseline. If progress has been made, students should determine if it is adequate given the timeline set in the original goal. If so, the student will continue implementation of the action plan.

If the student determines he is making progress but is not on course to meet the deadlines established in the goal, he should reconsider the frequency, duration, or intensity in which he is involved with or engaged in the action or strategies set in the goal.

If the student determines that she has not made any progress toward the goal or if she has readjusted her action plan several times and still does not seem to be on track to complete the goal in a timely manner, then she will need to revisit the goal and adjust it accordingly. It may be that the goal was too broad or addressed an outcome that was too hard or too distant. In most cases, students will want to look at the objectives they developed and determine if one of those might be better, serving as an intermediary step between current status and the longer-term goal. Students may also just want to revise the timelines set. Whatever the action, the key is that the student use the information from the evaluation to adjust his or her plan or goal.

SUMMARY

Setting and achieving goals is at the heart of acting in a self-determined manner. There is sufficient evidence that students with learning disabilities and emotional or behavioral disorders achieve more positive community and achievement outcomes when involved in interventions that incorporate goal setting. A sufficient literature base documents the efficacy of goal setting with people with intellectual and developmental disabilities, but those studies are dated and not as focused on outcomes that are more relevant today. That said, research has begun to link goal setting with more positive outcomes for students with intellectual and developmental disabilities. There are a variety of steps to teaching goal setting and attainment. Sands and Doll (2005) provided seven principles of teaching goal setting to students with disabilities that sum up many of the activities in teaching goal setting. These seven principles are listed in Table 4.1 (p. 59).

TABLE 4.1. Application Principles for Teaching Goal Setting

Application Principle 1	At all grades, help students work towards goals that are so specific that students know immediately whether or not they have been met.
Application Principle 2	At all grades, assist students to set manageable goals that they are likely to reach within a defined time interval: a class period, day, week, month or semester.
Application Principle 3	At all grades, set or help students set goals that are somewhat more challenging than you expect them to achieve.
Application Principle 4	Set or help students set goals that make meaningful connections between their learning and their home and community lives.
Application Principle 5	Set or assist students in setting goals that describe the processes or strategies they will use to accomplish a task or create a product.
Application Principle 6	When students cannot set goals for their own learning, providing them with teacher-set goals is an effective substitute.
Application Principle 7	Plan classroom activities to provide students with opportunities to set their own goals for learning at least some of the time.

Note. Data from Sands and Doll (2005).

CHAPTER 5

Teaching Self-Advocacy

Promoting self-advocacy is an important component of promoting self-determination, particularly for students with intellectual and developmental disabilities, who may need these skills to enable them to pursue goals that are based on their preferences or to keep someone else from making decisions about and for them. Teaching students to become more self-advocating involves teaching them about their rights and responsibilities; to be assertive; to communicate effectively; to negotiate, compromise, and persuade; and to be effective leaders or team members.

WHAT IS SELF-ADVOCACY?

To self-advocate is, quite simply, to stand up for oneself and to advocate on one's own behalf. The term "self-advocate" has most often been used in the context of adults with intellectual disabilities, in reference to people who are involved in organized self-advocacy groups or, less specifically, to adults who are more self-determined and more independent. Hayden and Nelis (2002) noted that self-advocacy has roots in all of the most recent social activist movements, including the women's suffrage movement of the 1910s and 1920s, the labor movement of the 1930s and 1940s, and the Civil Rights Movement of the 1950s and 1960s. The disability advocacy movement, which emerged in the 1970s and 1980s, emulated the earlier social activist movements, essentially resulting in a group of people with disabilities who had taken leadership in achieving greater civil liberties. This movement also spawned a system of self-advocacy organizations, consumer-organized and -controlled entities, for people with intellectual disabilities. These organizations, the first of which was People First of Oregon, founded in 1974, provided an important foundation to encourage individual and group advocacy for individuals with intellectual and developmental disabilities and to promote self-determination for those individuals. The founding of Self-Advocates Becoming Empowered (SABE) as a national association for self-advocacy organizations in 1991 provided a national focus for the self-advocacy movement. Currently, as a result of the disability advocacy movement and the growth of the national self-advocacy network, there is more participation of people with intellectual and developmental disabilities in national, state, and local policy development than probably at any time in history (Hayden & Nelis, 2002).

Is Self-Advocacy Important?

As noted in Chapter 1, self-determined people are causal agents in their own lives; they cause things to happen. They are goal-oriented and are able to take advantage of opportunities that move them closer to their goals. One does not achieve this, however, without, to some degree, advocating for oneself. For many students with disabilities, being passive is often easier than speaking up, and they are hesitant to seek the supports they need to achieve their goals.

A group of college students with disabilities participating in a summit called Aiming for the Future highlighted the importance of learning skills related to self-advocacy (Lehman, Davies, & Laurin, 2000). The purpose of the summit was to discuss barriers and needs related to postsecondary education, and the 35 college students participating identified the need to gain respect in the college community and to be more assertive in gaining knowledge. The students identified barriers to success as including lack of understanding and acceptance, lack of adequate services and financial resources, and lack of self-advocacy skills and training needed for independent living.

TEACHING SELF-ADVOCACY SKILLS

West and colleagues (1992) suggested that one way of teaching self-advocacy skills would be to have students role-play transition-related situations that would utilize self-advocacy skills, such as setting up their class schedule, moving out of the home, or meeting with a medical provider. Once students feel comfortable with specific self-advocacy skills and strategies, they should be encouraged to move beyond role playing. The educational and transition-planning process provides an ideal learning environment in which to put such skills into action, a topic dealt with in Chapter 11.

Another important way for students to learn self-advocacy skills is to become involved in organizations and clubs, both internal and external to the school system. There is an almost endless number of such outlets, from self-advocacy and self-help groups for people with disabilities to cause-related organizations like the Sierra Club, for example, to a fundraising campaign to build a local library. Students can identify their interests and abilities and become involved in activities that apply their leadership and self-advocacy skills in settings with others who share a common goal and who may provide support and encouragement.

Test, Fowler, Brewer, and Wood (2005) reviewed the extant literature pertaining to self-advocacy instruction for students with disabilities and suggested that teachers can use such techniques as role-playing, whole-group, small-group, or one-on-one instruction to implement self-advocacy instruction. Test and colleagues noted, however, that teachers need to examine their own cultural beliefs about student self-advocacy and investigate the cultural beliefs of their students' families to promote effective student involvement in self-advocacy during the school years (Test et al., 2005).

One model for self-advocacy aimed at middle school students utilized a portfolio system (Battle, Dickens-Wright, & Murphy, 1998). Kling (2000) weaves a number of self-advocacy skills into her ASSERT strategy, focused on children of all ages to support disability awareness and communication about disability. Steps in the ASSERT process are: *A*wareness of disability, *S*tate disability, *S*tate strengths and limitations, *E*valuate problem and solutions, *R*ole-play solution, and *T*ry it in the real setting. The approach focuses on disability awareness and self-advocacy related to self-disclosure of disability for students from early childhood to high school.

Teaching Assertiveness

To "assert" oneself means to act boldly, typically in stating or defending an opinion, or to defend one's rights. Rich and Schroeder (1976) defined assertive behavior as "the skills to seek, maintain, or enhance reinforcement in an interpersonal situation through the expression of feelings or wants when such expression risks loss of reinforcement or even punishment" (p. 1082).

Rakos (1991) identified several performance implications in this definition. First, the definition identifies assertiveness as a learned skill and as a function of the situation and the interaction of the person and situation. Second, the definition makes clear that "assertion is an expressive skill, composed of verbal and nonverbal response components and performed in an interpersonal context in which there is some risk of negative reaction by the recipient" (Rakos, 1991, p. 10). Finally, Rakos noted that assertiveness is both defined and measured by outcomes of the behavior.

Research has indicated that there are overt (e.g., observable) and covert (e.g., nonobservable) components of assertive behavior. Rakos (1991, p. 25) proposed three categories for overt response components of assertive behavior, which constitute the class of behaviors to be taught:

1. *Content*: the verbal behavior of the asserter, or what the asserter says to the other person(s).
2. *Paralinguistic elements*: the vocal characteristics of the verbal behavior, or how the asserter sounds.
3. *Nonverbal behaviors*: the body movements and facial expressions that accompany the verbal behavior, or how the asserter appears.

The content of assertive behaviors reflects two response categories: the expression of rights and the expression of elaborations. Elaborations are the "extra" aspects of the content that are part of successful assertive communication. Examples of these extras include explanations as to why one is expressing a specific right, an acknowledgment of the feelings or rights of the other person, compromises and alternatives, and, in some circumstances, apologies.

The expression of rights is, according to Rakos, the core of any assertion. The content of an assertion will contain a verbalization of desire, affect, or opinion. Rakos (1991, p. 72) proposed that the expression of rights can take several forms, including:

- Refusals (No thank you, I am not interested in contributing at this time).
- Behavior change requests (I would like you to _____).
- Expression of an unpopular or different opinion (I disagree with _____).

Students with intellectual and developmental disabilities will vary in the degree to which they need instruction in expressing rights or in employing elaborations. Some students may be perfectly capable of expressing their opinions, wants, or needs, yet have very limited skills using appropriate elaborations so that they can achieve their desired outcome. Other students may have limited experience with and opportunity to express their needs and may need instruction in that area.

The term "Paralinguistic elements" refers to the verbal characteristics of assertive behaviors. Instruction focuses on topics like voice characteristics (how loud or soft the assertion is made [e.g., voice volume], voice intonation and inflection, voice firmness) and characteristics of the response, including duration and fluency. Finally, "nonverbal behaviors" include eye contact, facial expressions, gestures, and body language. Students with disabilities typically can benefit from instruction in both paralinguistic and nonverbal components of assertive behavior.

Rakos (1991) also identified process skills that affect the success of assertive behaviors, such as response timing, or the degree to which a person responds to the situational cues in the interaction. Unskilled or inexperienced individuals fail to time their vocalizations and gestures, leaving long periods of silence or responding too quickly (Rakos, 1991). The degree to which someone both initiates an assertive behavior and persists in actions to achieve a desired outcome is also important to the relative success of the interaction.

Fujiki and Brinton (1993) and Brinton and Fujiki (1993) conducted two studies showing that people with intellectual disabilities were able to learn to become more assertive. Domingo, Barrow, and Amato (1998) found that adults with intellectual disabilities could learn communication skills that enabled them to exert control in their environment. Further, research by Hickson, Khemka, and colleagues (Hickson & Khemka, 1999; Khemka, 2000; Khemka & Hickson, 2000; Khemka, Hickson, & Reynolds, 2005), which is covered in Chapter 3, incorporates an assertiveness-training component to teach people with intellectual disabilities how to respond in situations of potential domestic abuse. In short, there is evidence that people with intellectual disabilities can acquire and use assertiveness skills.

Assertiveness Training

Assertiveness training originated with the work of Wolpe (Wolpe, 1969; Wolpe & Lazarus, 1966) and Salter (1949) and quickly became one of the most widely used treatments to promote assertive behavior (Rakos, 1991). The term "assertiveness training" has been applied to several intervention programs that share similar procedures (Rimm & Masters, 1979). Roffman (1994) summarized the basic elements of this approach as including (1) modeling, (2) behavior rehearsal, (3) reinforcement, (4) feedback and coaching, (5) positive self-statement training, (6) relaxation training, and (7) homework assignments.

Assertiveness training has been widely used and its efficacy documented both in the general population and in targeted populations, including people with substance abuse problems, depression, anxiety disorders, and other psychiatric disorders, as well as with populations defined by demographic characteristics (e.g., women, children, elderly people) (Rakos, 1991).

There has also been some research on assertiveness training and people with intellectual disabilities. Bates (1980) conducted weekly group social skills–training sessions with adults with intellectual disabilities. The training strategies followed the assertiveness-training model and included modeling, behavior rehearsal, coaching, structured feedback, contingent incentives, and homework assignments. Participants acquired each of the social skills successfully. Kirkland and Caughlin-Carver (1982) recruited 28 adults with intellectual disabilities to examine the efficacy of assertiveness training with this population. Participants were randomly assigned to an experimental or a control group. The experimental group received assertiveness training and was judged (based on ratings of videotaped role-play responses to specific problem situations) to be more assertive than the control group. Participants in the control group then received assertiveness training and showed significant improvement in their assertiveness skills. Bregman (1984) used assertiveness training with 128 adults with intellectual disabilities, with participants showing enhanced assertiveness skills and a more internal locus of control.

Assessing and Teaching Discrete Assertiveness Skills

While the most common approach identified in the literature to teach assertive behavior is assertiveness training, there are circumstances in which it may be more appropriate to focus on individual skill areas and teach these skills using another

TABLE 5.1. Skills Needed for Assertive Behavior

Skill area	Discrete skills
Expression of rights	• Identifies and articulates rights. • Identifies and articulates associated responsibilities. • Discriminates conflicts between rights of individual(s) and rights of groups. • Identifies and articulates personal beliefs and values. • Identifies and articulates differences among assertive, nonassertive, and aggressive behavior. • Discriminates among statements of wants, needs, opinion, and fact. • Understands inherent risk factor in assertion.
Verbal assertion skills	• Expresses rights statement in brief and direct manner. • Communicates rights statement in first person. • Discriminates between and employs refusals and behavior change requests. • Communicates opinions and beliefs appropriately. • Employs appropriate tone of voice. • Uses intonation and timing effectively. • Responds appropriately to aggression and persists in assertion.
Nonverbal assertion skills	• Uses and understands body language. • Uses gestures and facial expressions appropriately. • Makes eye contact appropriately. • Uses appropriate posture and body positioning.
Expression of elaborations	• Communicates understanding of others' feelings, opinions, or experiences. • Employs negotiation, compromise, and persuasion skills. • Modulates voice characteristics to match elaboration.
Conversation skills	• Practices active listening skills.

strategy instead of implementing the assertiveness-training approach in totality. Some students may already be competent in most skill areas related to assertive behavior and require instruction in one area only. Table 5.1 provides a list of some assertive behavior skills. The identification of target assertive behavior skills for intervention purposes involves a combination of assessment strategies, including the following.

Observation of Naturally Occurring Behavior

Perhaps the simplest assessment procedure, and the logical first step, is to observe a student's behavior in situations where opportunities to display assertive behavior are available. It is advisable to code these observations in some manner, either through longhand records, event recording, or behavioral counts. Such observations can form the basis for developing behavioral checklists, which can be used both to code future natural observations and to create teacher, parent, and student self-report checklists.

Completing Behavioral Checklists

Another means of gathering information about assertiveness is to complete behavioral checklists. Such lists of assertive behavior can be generated from observations or compiled from behaviors reported in the literature. Items should be worded in an active voice (e.g., ____ makes eye contact with other person). In addition to using checklists as coding sheets for observations, such lists can be completed by the teacher, student, and his or her family members.

Role-Play Assessments

One drawback to observations in natural settings is that the opportunities to observe students interacting in an assertive manner are relatively limited within the school. In addition, the presence of an observer in specific settings can alter behavior. One alternative is to develop role-play scenarios where students respond to a scripted problem situation. Teachers can identify areas of strengths and limitations across settings in which assertive behavior would be used.

Self-Monitoring

Student self-monitoring of behavior can be both an effective assessment tool and an intervention strategy. Teachers can work with students to identify assertive behaviors and ask students to monitor and in some manner record when they use such behaviors. It is prudent not to use self-monitoring as the sole assessment strategy, as having students attend to specific behaviors will probably increase the likelihood that they will perform those behaviors.

There are other assessment strategies, including sociometric ratings (e.g., asking classmates and peers to identify students who are assertive), standardized self-report measures, and analogue assessments (situations in which a student will need to be assertive are contrived within the typical environment). It is likely that educators will need to employ more than one of these methods in order to determine which behaviors warrant instructional intervention.

There are numerous examples in the literature providing an evidence base for teaching discrete skills related to assertiveness to students with intellectual disabilities (Bornstein, Bach, McFall, Friman, & Lyons, 1980; Senatore, Matson, & Kazdin, 1982; Korinek & Polloway, 1993).

Assertive, Nonassertive, and Aggressive Behaviors

Most strategies to promote assertive behavior teach students to discriminate among assertive, nonassertive, and aggressive behaviors and to express their wants, needs, or feelings in an assertive, not aggressive, manner. Aggressive behavior is behavior that is hostile and intended to hurt another person, but it is inappropriate to charac-

TABLE 5.2. Outcomes of Assertive, Nonassertive, and Aggressive Responses

Type of response	Outcome of response
Assertive	• Communicates knowledge of individual rights. • Acknowledges rights of others and value of those rights. • Enhances mutual respect. • Minimizes potential conflict. • Leads to enhanced self-confidence, internal control.
Nonassertive	• Fails to communicate rights message. • Invites others to take advantage of individual. • Limits potential for achieving desired outcome. • Completely avoids conflict.
Aggressive	• May hurt others and damage potential for collaboration and compromise. • Elicits defensive reactions and positioning. • Provides opportunity for temporary release of anger. • Limits potential for achieving desired outcome.

terize aggressive or nonassertive behaviors as always bad and assertive behaviors as always good. Students should be taught to recognize that, while there are occasions in which nonassertive or aggressive behaviors are more appropriate, these actions are typically less helpful options to achieve their desired outcomes.

One way to communicate the differences among assertive, nonassertive, and aggressive behaviors is to discuss the outcomes of each type of behavior, as illustrated in Table 5.2. Using strategies like role playing, it is easy to illustrate the differences among these three response classes and to highlight the outcomes associated with each. It is important to emphasize that acting assertively does have a risk factor. For example, whenever a person expresses his or her opinion or belief or requests that someone else change his or her behavior, there is the risk that others will disagree, become upset, or act aggressively in response. A nonassertive response in a situation might minimize the potential for disagreement or conflict at the risk of not achieving the desired outcome, but if a person is fairly certain that his or her assertive behavior will result in problems created by aggressive responses, he or she may choose a nonassertive course of action. Behaving assertively involves a constant evaluation of the risks and benefits of acting in an assertive manner.

Teaching Rights and Responsibilities

Since a rights expression is the core element of any assertive behavior, it stands to reason that students with disabilities should learn about rights and identify the responsibilities that accompany them. Strategies to teach assertive behavior focus on teaching students *how* to be assertive. Instruction in rights and responsibilities focuses on *what* to advocate or assert.

Many times, instruction on rights focuses solely on citizenship training—for example, voting skills, understanding the Constitution, and knowledge of laws

TABLE 5.3. Sample List of Basic Human Rights

- I have the right to state my opinions and my feelings.
- I have the right to refuse requests.
- I have the right to make my own decisions.
- I have the right to decide what to do with my property and time.
- I have the right to ask for information.
- I have the right to make choices based on my beliefs, values, and interests.
- I have the right to be treated with dignity and respect.
- I have the right to stand up for my own needs.
- I have the right to be listened to and taken seriously.
- I have the right to be alone when I wish.
- I have the right to a free, appropriate education.

Note. From Wehmeyer, Agran, and Hughes (1998). Copyright 1998 by Michael Wehmeyer, Martin Agran, and Carolyn Hughes. Reprinted by permission.

and the legislative process. While issues important in citizenship training certainly overlap with assertiveness training and effective communication, it is probably more important to the promotion of assertiveness to focus instruction on basic human rights and building the confidence to assert those rights.

The identification of basic human rights is, in many ways, an individual process. Certainly, governmental bodies have enunciated legally protected rights, and pseudogovernmental bodies such as the United Nations have declarations of basic human rights; however, in our society, there are also many rights that may be generally accepted but not civilly protected. In many cases, the need to be assertive relates to these nonprotected rights.

Teaching students to identify the basic human rights that are important to them begins with an understanding of civilly protected rights and expands to those rights that are important to the student based on his or her beliefs and values and the student's cultural environment. Table 5.3 provides a list of basic human rights.

Students need to understand further that rights are coupled with responsibilities and that others have rights that may, in some ways, conflict with their rights. Students should understand that just because they have a certain right or view something as a right does not give them a free ticket to do as they please or mean that others will recognize that right. It is for this reason that skills like negotiation and compromise, effective elaboration (e.g., acknowledging others' rights), and effective verbal and nonverbal communication are important.

TEACHING EFFECTIVE COMMUNICATION SKILLS

Throughout the previous section, we stressed the importance of effective communication skills to assertive behaviors. Effective communication skills are, in and of themselves, important skills for self-advocacy. These skills include conversation skills, listening skills, and body language skills. This section will describe the types of communication skills that warrant attention in self-advocacy instruction.

Conversation Skills

We have already discussed the importance of voice tone, volume, intonation, and inflection in assertive communication exchanges. These skills are equally important within the context of learning effective conversation skills. Understanding the dynamics of conversations can be important for students effectively to achieve the outcomes targeted by self-advocacy efforts. In addition to the nonverbal components of conversations and the paralinguistic aspects discussed previously, effective conversation skills include responding to a conversation partner's question or statement with a relevant statement or answer, initiating conversations at appropriate times, taking turns appropriately, and showing continued interest in a conversation by employing brief speech acknowledgers (e.g., "yes, I see" or "right"). Ineffective conversation skills include frequent silences following a conversation partner's questions or statements; short, abrupt responses; frequent interruptions; off-topic responses; inappropriate tone (e.g., a joke in response to a concern or problem); and mumbling or otherwise unintelligible responses.

The literature pertaining to teaching conversation skills is quite extensive, and we will not try to cover it. For example, Mattie (2001) taught adults with intellectual disabilities conversation skills using task analysis and cognitive training strategies. Hughes, Harmer, Killian, and Niarhos (1995) used self-instruction strategies to teach students with intellectual and developmental disabilities conversation skills in the context of their high school classrooms, and Hunt, Alwell, and Goetz (1991) taught students with severe disabilities to engage in conversational exchanges with friends and family.

Nonverbal Communication Skills

Nonverbal behaviors, like eye contact, facial expressions, gestures, and body language, are important components of communicative interactions. Students with intellectual and developmental disabilities often have difficulty interpreting these signals, and it is important to ensure that instruction includes these components of communication.

Active Listening

Listening to what is being said, rather than just talking (without listening), is a key element for those teaching self-advocacy to emphasize. Students should learn that listening skills may be as important to self-advocacy as assertiveness or conversation skills. Although students spend a great deal of time listening in educational settings, they often do not do so effectively. The same is true in conversations and other circumstances where communication is important.

Active listening is a strategy that has been employed to enhance listening skills in circumstances where self-advocacy skills might be employed. Instruction in active listening techniques asks students to:

1. *Look at the person who is speaking*. Stress that when someone looks at a person while that person is speaking, it tells the speaker that he or she is listening.
2. *Ask questions*. Emphasize that when a person is actively listening, the speaker is likely to say something that he or she can ask a question about. Questions can clarify something the speaker has said or confirm the speaker's statement. In both cases, the listener can gather more information and, at the same time, let the speaker know that he or she is listening.
3. *Don't interrupt*. While it is a good idea to ask some questions to show that one is listening, it is a bad idea to interrupt the speaker continually. A good listener lets another person speak without interrupting unless it is really necessary. Repeated interruptions send a message to the speaker that the listener does not really want to hear what he or she has to say.
4. *Take notes*. In some circumstances, it is appropriate to take notes. Note taking can help the listener remember what he or she learned in the conversation and, once more, lets the speaker know that he or she is listening.

TEACHING LEADERSHIP AND TEAMWORK SKILLS

Abery, Smith, Sharpe, and Chelberg (1995) suggested that most people, with or without a disability, do not view themselves as leaders, in part because of the images of leaders in our society. Leaders, contend Abery and colleagues (1995), are "viewed as charismatic individuals who inspire others to action through fiery speeches. Leaders are thought of as unusually attractive, intelligent, powerful, talented and/or prosperous. Still others think of leaders as martyrs who sacrifice all for a cause" (p. 1).

At least in part because of this view of leaders in our society, people with disabilities are rarely perceived as leaders (Abery et al., 1995; Wehmeyer & Berkobien, 1996). Disability and leadership are, in fact, often viewed as mutually exclusive. Stereotypes to the contrary, most people probably have the capacity to become leaders if one examines more closely what it means to lead. Leaders guide or direct others on a course of action, influence the opinions and behaviors of others, and show the way by going in advance. Leadership can take many forms, and many leaders do not fit the stereotypes. As such, the types of skills that leaders need to possess are varied and, in most cases, redundant to skills discussed in this chapter as well as in Chapters 3 and 4.

While skills development is an important part of learning to be a leader, it is also important that students have opportunities to learn to lead by leading. The educational planning process is an ideal venue in which to teach leadership skills and to provide opportunities for students to assume some leadership responsibilities, as discussed in Chapter 11. Specific skills instruction to promote leadership focuses on individual skills components, such as teaching students how to set goals, resolve conflicts, be assertive, foster teamwork and participation, communicate effectively, or run a meeting, all of which are dealt with in other chapters.

Students need to learn both to be effective team members and participants and, in the role of leader, to facilitate teamwork and participation. The goal of teamwork building is to get all participants working together to achieve a common objective or goal. The goal of participation skills building is to get each individual involved and contributing. Participation skills usually focus on the individual's ability to contribute to the discussion and the decision-making/problem-solving process as a whole. Thus, teaching students to be more effective decision makers or problem solvers will increase their participation skills. A frequently mentioned participation skill is the ability to critique ideas, proposals, and outcomes in a constructive manner. Effective critiquing skills develop as individuals have more opportunities to participate. There are also instructional activities that can promote the emergence of these skills. For example, Balcazar, Seekins, Fawcett, and Hopkins (1990) taught members of a self-help organization how to identify and report on disability-related issues to the whole group. Training included teaching members (1) how to identify disability-related issues from various sources; (2) how to report, evaluate, and critique a particular issue or practice; and (3) how to present this information to the group. This instruction included some role-playing and self-directed learning activities.

Conflict Resolution Skills

One of the more difficult challenges to teamwork that a leader must address is conflict in a group. Guerra, Moore, and Slaby (1995) provided a series of steps students could learn in a self-directed manner that would enable them to resolve conflicts.

1. *Why is there a conflict? Checking facts and beliefs.* In this step, students learn the importance of obtaining the factual information necessary to resolve the conflict and to explore their own beliefs about a situation. Guerra and colleagues (1995) stressed the importance of teaching students to look out for their own and others' biases in this step.
2. *Why is there a conflict? The perspective of others.* Students need to learn to think about a conflict situation from the perspective of all parties in order to craft a response that will resolve the conflict to the satisfaction of everyone involved.
3. *Thinking of solutions.* Based on the information gathered in the previous two steps, students need to learn to generate possible solutions to the problem. Guerra and colleagues (1995) stress using effective assertiveness and involving all parties in the generation of solutions.

4. *Deciding on a solution.* Students should apply decision-making skills to identify the most satisfactory solution to the conflict. At this point in the process, students will need to employ effective negotiation, compromise, and persuasion skills as well.
5. *Evaluate results.* Once a conflict has been resolved, students need to learn to monitor ongoing interactions and keep a similar situation from arising again.

Obviously, teaching conflict resolution skills involves teaching effective problem-solving skills, and these are discussed in depth in Chapter 3.

SUMMARY

Advocacy and self-advocacy skills are necessary for students, especially students with intellectual and developmental disabilities. Knowing what you want, knowing how to ask for it, and making sure your rights are honored are important elements of being self-determined. Educators and family members need to continue to encourage children and youth with disabilities to develop communication skills such as planning what to say, delivering the message in a way that is assertive (but not aggressive), and being able to negotiate and compromise when necessary. Students must understand how their disability affects their ability to communicate, the strengths and limitations they possess, and the rights and responsibilities that exist within the school, home, or community. Teachers and other adults should make sure that opportunities are present at home, at school, and in the wider community to express opinions and provide ongoing practice for students to speak up for themselves and others.

PART III

PROMOTING SELF-DETERMINED LEARNING

CHAPTER 6

Antecedent Event Regulation

An important focus in promoting self-determination is to enable students with intellectual and developmental disabilities to self-determine their learning. Chapters 6, 7, and 8 discuss student-directed learning strategies that enable students to become the causal agent in their learning, to become self-determined learners. We begin this chapter with a brief discussion of what we mean by "student-directed" and "self-determined" learning and the role of educators in self-determined learning.

STUDENT-DIRECTED LEARNING STRATEGIES AND SELF-DETERMINED LEARNING

Student-directed learning strategies enable students to modify and regulate their own behavior (Agran, King-Sears, Wehmeyer, & Copeland, 2003). The emphasis in such strategies is shifted from teacher-mediated and -directed instruction to student-directed instruction. By "student-directed," we mean that the student is an active participant in the instructional process. There are multiple benefits to implementing student-directed strategies; for example, teaching students to self-regulate learning enhances generalization. Further, student-directed learning promotes student self-determination.

Particularly for students with intellectual and developmental disabilities, student-directed and self-determined learning should not be confused with students learning without support. The intent in teaching students to self-direct learning is to maximize the degree to which students are causal agents in their learning. The teacher's role shifts from providing direct instruction to facilitating the learning process and providing whatever supports a student needs to succeed. Some students with more significant cognitive disabilities may need considerable scaffolding and support to implement student-directed learning strategies. The goal for such efforts is not complete independence, but to shift the focus from teacher-mediated and teacher-directed learning to student-directed activities. Students' use of self-directed learning strategies enables them to engage in what we have referred to as "self-determined learning" (Mithaug, Mithaug, Agran, Martin, & Wehmeyer, 2003). Chapter 9 provides a comprehensive instructional model to promote self-determined learning.

The most frequently identified student-directed learning strategies involve antecedent cue regulation, self-monitoring, self-evaluation, self-reinforcement, and self-instruction. This chapter focuses on teaching students antecedent event regulation (including antecedent cue regulation). Chapter 7 focuses on consequent event regulation (self-monitoring, self-evaluation, and self-reinforcement), and Chapter 8 focuses on teaching students self-instruction strategies.

Learners who self-determine learning know how to choose, act, and react to results in order to learn from choices they make within the learning process. This chapter and Chapter 7 describe how self-regulation of the antecedent and consequent events of learning leads to self-determined learning. This chapter describes key student-directed learning strategies to help learners regulate antecedents of learning, while Chapter 7 describes key student-directed learning strategies to help learners regulate consequences of self-engaged pursuits. Our central argument is that teaching students to regulate the antecedents and consequences of learning leads to maximizing achievement and its generalization across settings and time.

This chapter shows how the antecedent–consequent model used to illustrate an operant analysis of behavior also illustrates a self-regulation analysis, then shows how learners develop the capacity to choose opportunities to engage, choose expectations for learning something from those opportunities, and choose plans for meeting those expectations. Finally, this chapter summarizes the results of antecedent event regulation, which match (1) needs, interests, and abilities and opportunities to learn; (2) expectations for gain and opportunities to learn; and (3) plans of action and expectations for gain. When learners master these strategies, they have regulatory control over the antecedents of their learning.

THEORETICAL BASIS FOR ANTECEDENT EVENT REGULATION

Antecedent event regulation strategies teach students to use behaviors that serve as the discriminative stimulus to elicit or prompt the desired response or behavior from a student. This sounds more complex than it is. A common strategy, for example, involves picture prompts, which present visual representations of the steps in a task sequence to cue or prompt the student to go through the sequence.

Two Models of Antecedent and Consequent Control

Antecedent (and consequent) event regulation strategies derive from two theoretical sources, applied behavior analysis and self-regulation theory. Techniques in applied behavior analysis are based on the "three-term contingency" outlined by operant psychology. This phrase refers to the three components of every behavioral action, according to behavior analysts: the discriminative stimulus (S^D), the response, and the reinforcer or consequence. The discriminative stimulus is a specific event or environmental condition that serves as the stimulus to bring out the desired response. This stimulus is said to acquire control over the desired response when the response is paired with a reinforcer. A common discriminative stimulus is a teacher instruction or prompt a student to perform a task. The response is the behavior the student performs when presented the discriminative stimulus (i.e., the behavior the teacher is trying to teach the student). The reinforcer, or reinforcing stimulus (S^R), is an event or action that follows the response and increases the possibility that the response will be exhibited again. Whitman (1990) defined self-regulation as "a complex response system that enables individuals to examine their environments and their repertoires of responses for coping with those environments to make decisions about how to act, to act, to evaluate the desirability of the outcomes of the action, and to revise their plans as necessary" (p. 373).

Both operant and self-regulation models of control are similar in that they claim learning is a function of associations among antecedent events, behavior, and consequent events. According to the operant analysis of learning, when S^R follow responses that in turn follow antecedent events (S^D), an association occurs between S^D and the response. According to the self-regulation analysis of learning, when choice opportunities elicit responses that, in turn, produce adjustments or reactions to results, an association occurs between the choice opportunity and the learner's adjustment to it, and that association is what is learned or acquired.

The models differ, however, on the agency responsible for establishing those associations, as Figure 6.1 shows. According to operant analysis, an external agent—a teacher or the environment—is responsible for the association among the antecedent event, a behavior or response, and its consequences; according to self-regulation analysis, learners are agents of control. They choose the opportunities they will engage in, the gain they expect from their engagement, and how they will produce that gain. They also choose the consequences of those choices through their reactions. They choose responses that match plans, outcomes that evaluate actions, and adjustments based on those evaluations. When learners control both the antecedents and consequences of learning, they exhibit self-determined learning (Mithaug et al., 2003). We will now discuss antecedent event regulation strategies derived principally from applied behavior analysis, then continue with antecedent event regulation strategies derived from self-regulation theory.

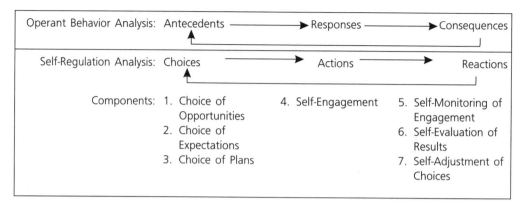

FIGURE 6.1. Comparing operant behavior analysis with self-regulation analysis.

ANTECEDENT CUE REGULATION AND PICTURE PROMPTS

"Antecedent cue regulation" refers to providing or making more noticeable a cue that results in a student initiating a desired behavior (Agran et al., 2003). When using an antecedent cue regulation strategy, the teacher provides a cue to prompt the student to begin a desired behavior. The types of antecedent cues that are presented vary considerably, but the most commonly used is picture prompts. Picture prompts are photographs, line drawings, or other graphics that illustrate the steps within a task sequence. Students use these visual cues to prompt or remind themselves to perform each component of a task or activity. The use of picture prompts has a long history of efficacy with students with intellectual and developmental disabilities. For example, Hughes and colleagues (2000) taught general education peer partners to teach high school students with severe intellectual disabilities to initiate conversations with their general education classmates in several settings, such as a physical education class, using a picture prompt system. Students with disabilities carried a small booklet containing line drawings that represented conversation topics. Peer partners taught students to look at a line drawing and ask their classmates a question related to the drawing. As the conversation progressed, students continued to turn the pages of the booklet, using the line drawings to cue them to ask additional questions.

Auditory cues are also effective. Taber-Doughty (2005) showed that students with intellectual and developmental disabilities could use either a picture prompt system or an audio prompt system to learn to operate office equipment. The audio prompts were provided by an MP3 player and the picture prompts provided through digital photographs. Chapter 10 provides information on the use of technology, including palmtop PCs, to deliver audio and video prompts.

Teaching Antecedent Cue Regulation

Agran and colleagues (2003) suggested steps for designing picture or audio prompt systems. The steps for a visual prompt system are:

1. Select a target task or routine.
2. Break the task or routine into substeps.
3. Select a type of visual prompt.
4. Create a visual prompt for each substep.
5. Decide how the picture prompts will be displayed.
6. Decide how the student will access or refer to the picture prompts.

The steps for an audio prompt system are:

1. Select a target task or routine.
2. Break the task or routine into substeps.
3. Write a script.
4. Record the script.
5. Determine how the recorded script will be delivered.

Of course, with technologies such as palmtop PCs, MP3 players, and other portable devices, video and audio prompts can be provided simultaneously and, importantly, in a relatively unobtrusive manner.

ANTECEDENT EVENT REGULATION
AND SELF-DETERMINED LEARNING

Antecedent cue regulation is based on the three-term contingency of operant psychology and emphasizes teacher delivery of a prompt. Antecedent event regulation (which, along with consequent event regulation, leads to self-determined learning), focuses on student choice as the focus of the antecedent event. Students choose the learning opportunity in which they engage and choose goals and action plans. This section examines how student regulation of antecedent events pertaining to choice can lead to self-determined learning.

Choosing Learning Opportunities

One of the first steps to establishing self-determined learning is to allow learners to choose from an array of tasks or learning opportunities. This important step enables students to compare their needs, interests, and abilities with their learning options and helps them identify the best match for them. Indeed, when students have repeated experiences choosing learning opportunities, they discover for themselves the types of learning tasks they like and in which they can engage successfully. This discovery was demonstrated by Mithaug and Hanawalt (1978) with students with intellectual and developmental disabilities. Students chose tasks on which to work from pair combinations they had been routinely assigned and required to work on in the past. Mithaug and Hanawalt, 1978) demonstrated that when students were given repeated opportunities to choose from random task pairs, they consistently chose some tasks and not others. In a second study (Mithaug & Mar, 1980), the same learners demonstrated that they were choosing according to their preferences because they consistently adjusted their choices in order to work tasks they indicated they preferred in the first study. In other words, through repeated choosing and adjusting to choice, they exhibited consistent preferences for classroom tasks their teachers judged equally interesting.

Mithaug, Martin, Agran, Husch, and Rusch (1988) prescribed a similar procedure for persons with severe disabilities seeking supported employment, which Martin, Mithaug, Husch, Frazier, and Marshall (2003) later implemented in an employment program that served 234 adults with developmental disabilities, 113 with severe learning disabilities, 145 with chronic mental illnesses, 61 with traumatic brain injuries, 102 with physical disabilities, and 96 with other disabilities. During Martin, Mithaug, Husch, and colleagues' (2003) 10-year project, the individuals receiving job placement services expressed their preferences before and after each job visit and then compared the two sets of ratings to determine whether they were consistent and, hence, whether the individuals had discovered what they liked and could do. For example, before going to a job site, they expressed their preferences for work conditions, task requirements, and job environments. After experiencing work at the site, they expressed their preferences again. They repeated this cycle again and again until they had sampled enough jobs and work conditions to make consistent choices about what they liked and could do.

The structure of the forms used during these repeated choice-making comparisons is illustrated in Figure 6.2. Like the procedure used in the Mithaug and Hanawalt (1978) and Mithaug and Mar (1980) studies, the procedure used in Martin, Mithaug, Husch, and colleagues' (2003) study allowed supported employment consumers to choose, experience choice, adjust to the choice, and choose again until the job situation they chose consistently matched their interests and capabilities. Martin, Mithaug, Oliphant, Husch, and Frazier (2002) reported that those individuals who completed the choice process were significantly more likely to be employed in the jobs they chose. Moreover, 71% of completers with developmental

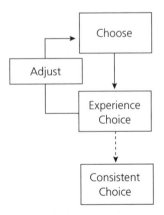

FIGURE 6.2. Reported choice during self-regulation.

disabilities found jobs that matched their first choice, 21% found jobs that matched their second choice, and 8% found jobs that matched their third choice.

Forms like the one in Figure 6.3 illustrate how study participants discovered for themselves the work conditions that they liked. First, they indicated on the form the work conditions they preferred. Then they visited the prospective job to determine whether those conditions were present. Finally, they compared their preferences with the conditions at the site and counted the number of matches to decide whether the job was a good fit for them.

Unfortunately, choice opportunities like these are often not available to students with intellectual and developmental disabilities, even in most efforts to promote self-determination. In a review of programmatic efforts to promote self-determination, Karvonen, Test, Wood, Browder, and Algozzine (2004) found that teachers were instructing students directly on what to choose:

> . . . once students were aware of the range of options, teachers engaged in discussions about the benefits, drawbacks, and potential long-term consequences of each decision. As one teacher pointed out,
>
> A lot of [how teachers promote self-determination] . . . is that ongoing engagement with students about, "this decision means this. This decision means that. This is what you need to do to prepare if this is where you're headed." And that is probably, one of the more powerful things in all of the structure that goes with that. (p. 33)

The problem with this type of instruction is that if students are to become self-determined learners, they need to learn to express preferences and adjust to their own choices.

Choosing Goals and Plans

Once a student has selected a learning task or opportunity, he or she must select a goal. As discussed in Chapter 7, addressing the discrepancy between one's current status and one's goal status is at the heart of self-regulation and self-determined learning. Students can use goal-setting strategies to help them choose outcomes to expect from the learning opportunities or tasks they have selected. Indeed, as covered in Chapter 4, there is evidence that having students engage in goal setting yields a wide range of adaptive benefits.

There is also substantial evidence of benefit from using forms and visual prompts or cues to present various types of schedules and menus for easy use in remembering school, employment, and community living choices to make (Agran, Fodor-Davis, Moore, & Deer, 1989; Irvine, Erickson, Singer, & Stahlberg, 1992; Martin, Elias-Burger, & Mithaug, 1987; Martin, Mithaug, & Frazier, 1992; Martin, Rusch, James, Decker, & Trtol, 1982). Mithaug and Mithaug (2003) compared two types of instruction to assess their effects on the independent work of young children with developmental disabilities. In one teaching condition, the teacher taught students to make choices on a self-regulation card (Figure 6.4) by instructing them

CHARACTERISTICS I LIKE VS. HERE FORM - A

NAME: JOB SITE:

DATE:

WHAT I LIKE (before work)		*	√	WHAT IS HERE (after work)		Matches	CHARACTERISTICS SUMMARY
Circle preferred. *Star top 10. √ 4 most preferred.				Circle the item that is here out of each pair.		Circle Y or N	
work alone	lots of people around			work alone	lots of people around	Y N	
quiet work-place	noisy workplace			quiet work-place	noisy workplace	Y N	
part time	full time			part time	full time	Y N	
weekdays only	weekends too			weekdays only	weekends too	Y N	
hard job	easy job			hard job	easy job	Y N	
work inside	work outside			work inside	work outside	Y N	
few rules	lot of rules			few rules	lot of rules	Y N	
standing up	sitting down			standing up	sitting down	Y N	
work mornings	work after-noons			work mornings	work after-noons	Y N	
attractive place	looks of place do not matter			attractive place	looks of place do not matter	Y N	
dress up for work	do not dress up			dress up for work	do not dress up	Y N	
physical work	thinking work			physical work	thinking work	Y N	
detail im-portant	detail not important			detail im-portant	detail not important	Y N	
job same every day	job different every day			job same every day	job different every day	Y N	
work with people	work with things			work with people	work with things	Y N	
important to work fast	not important to work fast			important to work fast	not important to work fast	Y N	
little super-vision	a lot of su-pervision			little super-vision	a lot of su-pervision	Y N	
daytime work	night work			daytime work	night work	Y N	
small business	big business			small business	big business	Y N	
other:				other:		Y N	
other:				other:		Y N	
other:				other:		Y N	

CHARACTERISTICS SUMMARY column notes:

job characteristics matches: _____

job characteristics matches available _____

= (_____ characteristics match)

characteristics match X 100 = _____ %
characteristics match

| not a 0% match | some 25% match | ok 50% match | good 75% match 100% |

Directions for determining the Most Important Characteristics Match:
After determining the top 4 charac-teristics and checking them, Place an OK beside each checked item that matches the same char-acteristic circled in the WHAT IS HERE column.

OK's = _____ X 100 = _____ %
4
Most Important Characteristics Match

FIGURE 6.3. Choosing work preferences for supported employment. From Martin, Mithaug, Oliphant, Husch, and Frazier (2002). Copyright 2002 by Paul H. Brookes. Reprinted by permission.

Is My Goal Reading?	What Will I Do in Reading?	What Did I Do in Reading?	Did I Match (Meet) My Goal?
	Read section in workbook	Read section in workbook	
Yes/No	Yes/No	Yes/No	Yes/No
Is My Goal Math?	What Will I Do in Math?	What Did I Do in Math?	Did I Match (Meet) My Goal?
	Complete math worksheet	Completed math worksheet	
	Yes/No		
Yes/No		Yes/No	Yes/No
Is My Goal Science?	What Will I Do in Science?	What Did I Do in Science?	Did I Match (Meet) My Goal?
	Complete science worksheet	Completed science worksheet	
Yes/No	Yes/No	Yes/No	Yes/No
Is My Goal Social Studies?	What Will I Do in Social Studies?	What Did I Do in Social Studies?	Did I Match (Meet) My Goal?
	Complete social studies worksheet	Completed social studies worksheet	
Yes/No	Yes/No	Yes/No	Yes/No
Is My Goal Writing?	What Will I Do in Writing?	What Did I Do in Writing?	Did I Match (Meet) My Goal?
	Write a journal entry	Wrote a journal entry	
Yes/No	Yes/No	Yes/No	Yes/No
		Number of Goals Met (Yesses)?	
		Number of Goals Set (Yesses) *Next Time*?	

FIGURE 6.4. Student self-regulation card.

what to circle on the card. In the other condition, she allowed students to learn about those choice options by making their own choices.

The two instructional approaches that immediately preceded students' independent use of the cards had significantly different effects on performance. For all students, assignment completion rates were higher when student-directed instruction immediately preceded independent work than when teacher-directed instruction preceded it. In other words, when students were allowed to choose during instruction, they were more likely to persist in use of their self-regulation cards during independent work. Apparently, telling students what to choose during instruction had a dampening effect on their independent choice making and follow-through.

Martin, Mithaug, Cox, and colleagues (2003) demonstrated the importance of giving students time to adjust and learn in a study involving eight secondary-age students with disabilities who used similar cards to self-regulate their work on various academic subjects throughout the day. In that study, students were free to use their cards throughout the school day to determine what to do, when to do it, what they accomplished, and what to adjust the next day for the same subjects. Martin, Mithaug, Cox, and colleagues (2003) reported that these students became significantly more proficient regulators over time in that they significantly increased the correspondence between their choices and actions, between their actions and evaluations, between their evaluations and adjustments, and between their adjustments and their next day's choices. Their performance in the academic subjects improved significantly as well. This result illustrates the relationship between antecedent event regulation and consequent event regulation, covered in Chapter 7.

Columbus and Mithaug (2003) used a similar set of forms to prompt 36 high school students with developmental disabilities to identify their needs and interests, set goals and develop plans to meet them, take action on these plans, evaluate the results, and then adjust goals and plans based on their evaluation. They then compared self-determination levels of a group that received self-regulation instruction with levels of a comparable group of students from the same school that used a self-report measure of self-determination. Prior to the instructional intervention, both groups reported equal levels of self-determination, but after instruction on use of the forms, the intervention group reported significantly higher levels of self-determination. Those students also reported more frequent expressions of their needs and interests, more frequent goal setting and making plans, and more frequent episodes of taking action on plans, evaluating results, and adjusting to their evaluations. The instructed group also reported more frequent opportunities for self-determined pursuits at home and at school.

The adults with severe disabilities who participated in the consumer-directed supported employment program described earlier (Martin et al., 2002) used a similar set of forms to choose, act, evaluate, and adjust their way to successful job performances once they got the job they wanted. They learned to self-regulate their work on the job using an array of picture-cued forms that guided them through choosing, working, evaluating, and adjusting. The forms they used were picture-cued because many could not read but could follow the cues sufficiently to make rational matches.

Figure 6.5 illustrates one of those forms. It helped consumers with intellectual and developmental disabilities adjust at their jobs by setting daily goals based on needs identified from the previous day's work. They completed the first two columns (e.g., "Goal," "How?") before they began work and the last three columns after they finished work. In the first two columns, they set their goals for the domains indicated in the rows and then indicated their plan for meeting each goal. After they finished work for the day, they completed the remaining columns. In the third column (e.g., evaluations), they assessed their performance and got their job coach's assessment of their day's performance and in the fourth column (e.g., "Match"), they indicated whether their assessment and their coach's agreed. In the last column (e.g., "Next"), they indicated whether they would work on the same

THE WORK IMPROVEMENT FORM - B

NAME: _____ JOB SITE: _____

DATE: _____ SESSION NO: _____

GOAL	HOW?	EVALUATIONS	great	MATCH?	NEXT
follow company rules	By _____	I Think ☐ Job Coach Thinks ☐ follow company rules / break rules ☐		YES / NO	follow company rules
come to work	By _____	I Think ☐ Job Coach Thinks ☐ come to work / miss work ☐		YES / NO	come to work
work safely	By _____	I Think ☐ Job Coach Thinks ☐ work safely / work unsafely ☐		YES / NO	work safely
listen & use feedback	By _____	I Think ☐ Job Coach Thinks ☐ listen & use feedback / reject feedback ☐		YES / NO	listen & use feedback
right pace for job	By _____	I Think ☐ Job Coach Thinks ☐ right pace for job / too fast/too slow ☐		YES / NO	right pace for job
take specified breaks	By _____	I Think ☐ Job Coach Thinks ☐ take specified breaks / not take specified breaks ☐		YES / NO	take specified breaks
work accurately	By _____	I Think ☐ Job Coach Thinks ☐ work accurately / make mistakes ☐		YES / NO	work accurately
come to work on time	By _____	I Think ☐ Job Coach Thinks ☐ come to work on time / come to work late ☐		YES / NO	come to work on time
attention to work	By _____	I Think ☐ Job Coach Thinks ☐ attention to work / distracted from work ☐		YES / NO	attention to work
if miss work, call	By _____	I Think ☐ Job Coach Thinks ☐ if miss work, call / miss work without calling ☐		YES / NO	if miss work, call

SUMMARY OF WORK ISSUES

matches with job coach _____ / # matches available _____ = work matches _____ X100= _____ % work matches

#job coach positives: _____ / #positives available _____ = work positives _____ X 100 = _____ % job coach work positives

0% not a match 25% some match 50% ok match 75% good match 100%

FIGURE 6.5. Sample work improvement contract. From Martin, Mithaug, Oliphant, Husch, and Frazier (2002). Copyright 2002 by Paul H. Brookes. Reprinted by permission.

goal the next day. With forms like this, these unlikely workers were able to get the information they needed, choose goals, make plans, evaluate themselves, and adjust from one day to the next.

Self-regulation forms like these were inspired in part by studies conducted in the 1980s that used similar forms to help underachieving elementary school students improve their performance on math problems. In those studies, students used the cards to set goals, work problems, evaluate results, and reinforce themselves for good work. The results were remarkable in that there were significant effects across all the possible generalization domains: subjects, behaviors, tasks, environments, and time (Stevenson & Fantuzzo, 1984, 1986). In our view, there were two reasons for the effects. First, students learned key self-regulation strategies needed to guide their independent study behaviors. Second, the self-regulation card provided prompts or cues reminding them where they were in the choice, work, evaluation, and adjustment process. Whether they were at home, at school, or somewhere else, the card was still present, guiding their choice of goals, their actions to meet their goals, their results to evaluate these actions, and their future goals and plans. The success of this simple yet direct approach to teaching self-determined behavior has yet to be duplicated by any other method of instruction.

SUMMARY

This chapter described a set of strategies that help learners self-regulate antecedent events that contribute to learning. The most commonly used antecedent event regulation strategies involve picture and audio prompts, and there is evidence that these strategies can enable students with intellectual and developmental disabilities to learn and perform tasks. This chapter also examined antecedent event regulation leading to self-determined learning. The strategies described help students answer questions that arise when confronted with a learning opportunity that may require a different way of responding: "Should I act?" "What will I get if I act?" "What should I do to get what I expect?" Most of us answer questions like these routinely, without much thought, but many students lacking basic self-regulatory competencies do not. For them, questions like these go unanswered mainly because they do not know what to do, and they avoid situations resulting in those questions. This chapter identified several straightforward approaches to helping these learners make choices and learn by adjusting repeatedly. These approaches are based on a vast body of research showing the benefits of using strategies for choosing opportunities, setting expectations, and planning behaviors that reduce the prospects for failure and increase the prospects for success. In the next chapter, we consider a companion set of strategies that helps learners regulate the consequences of engaging in new opportunities.

CHAPTER 7

Consequent Event Regulation

In Chapter 1, we reviewed theoretical models of self-determination that have been applied to the development of interventions to promote and enhance self-determination. Central to these models is the role of student self-regulation. But why do students engage in self-regulation? Mithaug (1993) suggested that individuals are often in flux between goal or desired states and existing or actual states. It is the acknowledgment of this discrepancy—the difference between what one has and what one wants—that provides the incentive for self-regulation and subsequent action. In this respect, self-regulation serves a problem-solving function. The first step in problem solving is to acknowledge that a problem exists. The individual then sets out to determine what ends or changes are or are not achievable. Regrettably, Mithaug (1993) noted, because of a fear of failure or a sense of powerlessness, people with disabilities often do little to change their situations and run into difficulties because they either avoid any action or set expectations that are too low or too high. Negative feelings about oneself produce lower expectations and confidence for the individual. Conversely, higher expectations result in more success and greater capacity in seeking out opportunity for gain.

To promote success, individuals need to enhance or increase their expectations. The ability to set appropriate expectations is based on the individual's success in matching his or her capacity with opportunity. "Capacity" is the individual's assessment of existing resources (e.g., work skill repertoire, knowledge about task requirements), and "opportunity" refers to the existing situation that will allow the individual to achieve the desired gain. Mithaug (1993) referred to optimal prospects as "just-right" matches. Such matches involve situations in which individuals are able correctly to match their capacity (skills, interests) with existing opportunities (e.g., potential jobs). The experience generated during self-regulation "is a function of repeated interaction between capacity and opportunity over time" (Mithaug, 1996, p. 159).

Another component of self-regulation is developing and using strategies for optimizing opportunity for gain, including self-management strategies that allow individuals to monitor, evaluate, and reinforce their own behavior and set their own goals. Yet another component of self-regulation is evaluating the effectiveness of a strategy and adjusting one's actions or the goal. Such adjustment involves repeating the procedure, changing the strategy, or changing the criterion level for the goal. In this chapter, we refer to the process of adjustment as consequent event regulation because one is adjusting one's actions as a function of the outcomes of the action taken.

Mithaug suggested that four factors determine the efficacy of self-regulation and, ultimately, the individual's success. These factors are past gain (previous success experiences), expectations for gain (just-right matches), choices, and actions (consequent event regulation). With additional experience in self-regulation, students can gain expertise in identifying short- and long-term goals, the resources and actions needed to achieve these goals, and self-corrective procedures if success eludes them.

In Chapter 6, we examined the role of antecedent event regulation in promoting self-determination and self-determined learning. This chapter will examine the consequent event regulation strategies that, along with antecedent event regulation strategies, lead to self-determined learning. Although goal setting is incorporated into the consequent event regulation process, because of its importance to self-determination we have discussed it in depth in Chapter 4. We conclude this chapter with a discussion of the contribution of consequent and antecedent event regulation to self-determination.

We begin with a discussion of the most frequently used student-directed learning strategies that make up the consequent event regulation process.

SELF-MONITORING

It is widely accepted that learning to monitor one's behavior is a prerequisite to self-regulation. Students who monitor their own behavior are better able to identify a discrepancy between an existing performance level and a future or desired level. In other words, it keeps us focused on our plan so that we do what we set out to do; it helps us match our behavior to our plan.

Self-monitoring involves a student's observation of his or her own behavior and recording whether a particular behavior occurred. Target behaviors may include practically any behavior the student (or teacher) wishes to modify. For example, Agran, Blanchard, Wehmeyer, and Hughes (2001) taught six secondary-level students with intellectual and developmental disabilities to monitor their use of several classroom study and organizational skills (e.g., recording and completing assignments, using a day planner). The students were instructed to place a tally mark on a card after they performed a target behavior. Dramatic improvements were reported for all students. Gilberts, Agran, Hughes, and Wehmeyer (2001) taught five middle school students with severe cognitive disabilities to monitor a set of classroom "survival" skills. These skills included being in class and in seat when the bell rang, having appropriate materials, greeting the teacher and other students, asking and answering questions, sitting up straight and looking at the teacher when addressed, acknowledging teacher and student comments, and using a planner. Positive changes were reported for all students, and the behaviors were maintained at 100%.

How important is accuracy relative to the student's self-monitoring? Interestingly, students who may not be accurate or honest in monitoring their behavior can still exhibit desirable behavior changes (Reinecke, Newman, & Meinberg, 1999). There is ample research to suggest that self-monitoring produces a reactive effect in which the student attends more to his or her behavior and, by doing so, provides stimuli to cue the appropriate response (Smith & Nelson, 1997) even when the self-monitoring is inaccurate. Consequently, the self-monitoring procedure may produce a desired effect without any other intervention (Agran & Martin, 1987). Nevertheless, it is wise to build in occasional teacher checks for accuracy, which may occur less frequently as the student becomes more proficient with self-monitoring.

The main reason for the strategy's pervasive effects, we would suggest, is that self-monitoring identifies or highlights various discrepancy conditions present in the adjustment process. It reveals discrepancies between what we want and what we have, what we seek to achieve and how we plan to achieve it, what we have done and what we had planned to do, what we hoped to get and what we have gotten, what we got and what we wanted to get. Once we are made aware of these conditions, we tend to act to eliminate them, which often improves adjustment.

SELF-EVALUATION

Self-evaluation involves the comparison of the behavior monitored to the student's desired goal or a teacher-determined standard. It is a critical self-regulation skill because it allows the student to become aware of whether he or she is meeting a desired goal and may potentially serve as a reinforcing event (Agran & Hughes, 1997). Self-evaluation extends self-monitoring methods from a frequency tally to an informed judgment and is usually paired with self-monitoring in its implementation. Self-evaluation provides the student with a standard against which to assess his or her behavioral performance (Agran, 1997). If the standard is met, the strategy may assume a reinforcing property, which will promote the likelihood of the behavior occurring in the future. If the standard is not met, the student is alerted to the apparent discrepancy between the desired performance level and the observed performance level. Of critical importance is the fact that the student provides him-

or herself with the feedback and is not dependent on a teacher or other individual to evaluate his or her behavior.

The advantages of self-evaluation are obvious. Teachers spend considerable time providing feedback to students. When students learn how to evaluate their own behavior, teachers can shift their attention to other responsibilities. Most important, students are not dependent on teachers to judge how well they are doing but, instead, learn how to evaluate their behavior and make changes toward improvement. The gains from this process are well supported in the self-regulation literature (Mithaug, Mithaug, Agran, Martin, & Wehmeyer, 2003).

Self-evaluation can be taught independently or as part of a total self-regulation approach, which typically involves goal setting, self-monitoring, and self-reinforcement. For example, middle school students with disabilities learned how to self-monitor their behavior during class and then self-evaluate their behavior at the end of class to increase their on-task behavior (Dalton, Martella, & Marchand-Martella, 1999). The students used the classroom clock as their cueing system to monitor work performance ("Are you working?") every 5 minutes. Also, they used a checklist noting specific classroom tasks (e.g., "Did you get your homework done?"), which also required a yes or no response. The checklist contained a series of questions for selected classroom behaviors required at the beginning of class ("Did you get started on time?"), during class ("Did you self-monitor to stay on task?"), and at the end of class ("Did you follow the teacher's directions?"). After completing the checklist, the students evaluated their behavior. The intervention increased students' on-task behavior and teachers' ratings of students' classroom behavior.

SELF-REINFORCEMENT

Self-reinforcement represents a major component of most conceptualizations of self-regulation. There is evidence to suggest that self-reinforcement is as effective, if not more effective, than teacher-delivered reinforcement. Self-reinforcement involves teaching students to reinforce themselves immediately after a desired behavior has occurred (Wehmeyer, Agran, & Hughes, 1998). Students are always present to administer their own consequences or feedback, so the possibility of lost reinforcement is minimized. Also, students normally may have difficulty acquiring desired outcomes because the available consequences are too delayed, too small, or not achievable. Self-reinforcement solves this potential problem in providing an opportunity for the student to reinforce him- or herself immediately (Malott, 1984). Traditionally, teachers have been in control of the consequences in a learning situation. Self-reinforcement shifts that control to the student, and it is this shift that provides considerable potency to student-determined learning.

Two activities are involved in self-reinforcement: discrimination and delivery. A student must discriminate that the target behavior has occurred before he or she can reinforce him- or herself (delivery). In this sense, self-reinforcement is functionally linked to self-monitoring. Similar to self-monitoring, self-reinforcement has stimulus properties that may cue appropriate responding.

Self-reinforcement is almost always used in conjunction with other strategies because information on matches between behavior and standards or results is necessary to justify rewards or reinforcers (Castro & Rachline, 1980; Hanel & Martin, 1980; Mahoney, Moura, & Wade, 1973; Martin & Hrydowy, 1989; Masters, 1968; Masters & Christy, 1974; Nelson & Birkimer, 1978; Shapiro, McGonigle, & Ollendick, 1980; Spates & Kanfer, 1977). It is possible that the changes in behavior attributed to self-reinforcement may, in fact, be due to the knowledge of results generated by self-monitoring and self-evaluation. It is also possible that this knowledge is in play even when self-reinforcement is studied alone because people are always free to self-monitor and self-evaluate covertly in order to regulate their behavior.

Still, researchers report positive results when the strategy is purported to be functioning independently, such as to control weight (Castro & Rachline, 1980; Mahoney et al. 1973), increase work of adults with intellectual disabilities (Hanel & Martin, 1980; Martin & Hrydowy, 1989), increase control of impulsivity (Nelson & Birkimer, 1978), and develop appropriate conversation skills in teenagers with autism (Newman, Buffington, & Hemmers, 1996).

Also of interest with regard to self-reinforcement is a body of research indicating that the agency of reward delivery—the self—can have an independent effect on the persistence of behavior (Agran et al., 2001; Barling & Patz, 1980; Dickerson & Creedon, 1981; Fantuzzo & Clement, 1981; Fredericksen & Fredericksen, 1975; Gettinger, 1985; Helland, Paluck, & Klein, 1976; Keogh, Whitman, & Maxwell, 1988; Lovitt & Curtiss, 1969). This finding is of interest because it is consistent with the more general proposition that when people choose which opportunities to engage in, they are more likely to persist in their engagement than when other people choose for them. Applied to the delivery of rewards, the same reasoning applies. When actors control the delivery of rewards, they are more likely to persist in their rewarded behavior than when other people control those deliveries.

CONSEQUENT EVENT REGULATION AND STUDENTS WITH INTELLECTUAL AND DEVELOPMENTAL DISABILITIES

Self-Monitoring

Self-monitoring is the most researched of the three major components of self-regulation and has yielded consistent results across a wide range of people and behaviors. It has been used to improve critical learning skills and classroom involvement skills of students with severe disabilities (Agran et al., 2005; Gilberts et al., 2001; Hughes et al., 2002), reading comprehension for students with learning disabilities (Jitendra, Hoppes, & Zin, 2000), writing performance for students with learning disabilities (Graham & Harris, 2005), performance in math for students with emotional disorders (Levendoski & Cartledge, 2000), and on-task behavior of students with autism (Coyle & Cole, 2004).

Some recent research has focused on the effects of self-monitoring on outcomes for students with intellectual and developmental disabilities. Hughes and colleagues (2002) used a multiple-baseline-across-participants design to examine the effects of self-monitoring on selected social and academic behaviors of high school students with intellectual disabilities who were enrolled in general education classes. Occurrences of self-monitoring were associated with improvement in target behaviors across participants. In addition, students' teachers and classmates perceived improved performance of target behaviors when students used their self-monitoring strategies. Copeland, Hughes, Agran, Wehmeyer, and Fowler (2002) used self-monitoring as a key element of a multicomponent intervention to improve academic performance of students with intellectual disabilities in general education classrooms. Use of self-monitoring improved performance on assignments for all participants and resulted in higher grades for three of four participants. Three of the participants also correctly and independently evaluated their performance in relation to their performance goals.

O'Reilly and colleagues (2002) taught a student with severe disabilities to self-monitor the occurrence of stereotyped behavior in a general education classroom. The student significantly increased his on-task behavior in the classroom while self-monitoring stereotyped behavior and decreased on-task behavior when the self-monitoring intervention was removed. Browder and Minarovic (2000) taught employees with intellectual disabilities who did not read to use sight words to self-initiate job tasks in competitive employment settings and incorporated a self-monitoring component into the intervention.

Self-Evaluation

The research literature on the efficacy of self-evaluation is substantial, although not as extensive as that on self-monitoring. To illustrate, consider this range of applications: work productivity of trainees with intellectual disabilities in a community-based restaurant training program (Grossi & Heward, 1998), disruptive behaviors of adolescents in a psychiatric hospital school (Kaufman & O'Leary, 1972), attention to task and academic productivity of students with learning disabilities (Lloyd, Hallahan, Kosiewicz, & Kneedler, 1982), increasing task mastery of young children (Masters, Furman, & Barden, 1977), increasing play skills of children (Nelson, Smith, & Colvin, 1995), increasing generalization and maintaining treatment gains of students with behavior problems during transitions from resource to regular classrooms (Rhode, Morgan, & Young, 1983), improving independent work skills of young children with disabilities (Sainato, Strain, Lefebvre, & Rapp, 1990), increasing on-task behavior of elementary school children (Thomas, 1976), and increasing homework completion of students with learning disabilities (Trammel, Schloss, & Alper, 1994).

In a study conducted by Agran, Blanchard, and Wehmeyer (2000), a student with intellectual disability and diabetes was taught to evaluate whether she had sufficient insulin in order to give herself the correct amount of insulin at lunchtime. This responsibility was based on the consequences of making an error. The goal was for the student to become 100% proficient in following the procedures outlined as anything less than that could have life-threatening consequences. The strategy proved successful. In this self-evaluation application, the student was literally given control over her own health and well-being.

In another application of self-evaluation, three adolescents with developmental disabilities were taught to evaluate their classroom behavior relative to goals they had initially set for themselves (Wehmeyer, Yeager, Wade, Agran, & Hughes, 2003). The target behaviors included improving their listening skills, not touching other students, increasing on-task behavior, and decreasing inappropriate verbalizations and disruptive behavior. The students compared their self-monitored recordings to those of a second observer to determine if they met the self-selected goal. Improvements in behavior were reported for all students.

Self-Reinforcement

Self-reinforcement occurs when actors reward themselves for accomplishing what they intend. It is almost always implemented with self-monitoring and/or self-evaluation procedures, so there are fewer studies that use this strategy exclusively. Wehmeyer and colleagues (2003) implemented self-reinforcement as part of a multicomponent intervention with students with intellectual disabilities in general education classrooms and found that the approach improved adaptive classroom behaviors and decreased maladaptive behaviors.

TEACHING SELF-MONITORING, SELF-EVALUATION, AND SELF-REINFORCEMENT

The first step in teaching self-monitoring is to teach the student to determine when he or she has correctly completed a task. Schloss and Smith (1998) suggested several steps:

1. Clearly define the behavior that will be self-monitored.
2. Explain the purpose of self-monitoring.
3. Model the self-monitoring strategy.
4. Practice with role play.

Agran, King-Sears, Wehmeyer, and Copeland (2003) suggested a four-step process to teach self-monitoring. A mnemonic, SPIN, represents the phases of the framework, and specific teacher tasks are identified for each phase:

- *S*elect the target behavior—(1) identify and define the behavior to be self-monitored, (2) measure current performance levels of the behavior, and (3) determine mastery criteria.
- *P*repare to teach self-monitoring—(1) determine the type of self-monitoring procedure, and (2) develop materials and lesson plans needed to teach self-monitoring.

- *Instruct the student using instructional process*—introduce the behavior to be self-monitored,
- *Note the student's performance*—(1) assess performance of the behavior, and (2) assess maintenance of the behavior.

Classroomwide self-monitoring systems can also be used. Kern, Dunlap, Childs, and Clarke (1994) taught students to self-monitor the following activities:

- I am on task.
- I had appropriate adult interactions.
- I had a positive attitude.

Students had recording sheets taped to their desks. When they heard a bell sound from a tape recorder, they responded to each of these statements. The bell was set for a variable 5-minute interval schedule across a 45-minute math period. The SPIN process used by Agran and colleagues (2003) can also be used to teach self-reinforcement and self-evaluation. These authors suggest that in the Instruct phase, there are three steps:

1. *Introduce the behavior to be self-evaluated or -reinforced.* Name the desired behavior and demonstrate examples and nonexamples. Discuss the benefits of the desired behavior. Provide practice of the desired behavior and name the mastery criteria.
2. *Introduce the self-evaluation or -reinforcement documentation device.* Describe self-evaluation or -reinforcement procedures and materials and strategy's benefits. Model the self-evaluation or -reinforcement procedure while performing the target behavior.
3. *Provide practice and assess mastery.* Provide guided practice for using self-evaluation or -reinforcement. Role-play desired behavior. Assess student's mastery of procedure within role-play situation. Discuss the specific situation in which self-evaluation or -reinforcement will be used. Provide independent practice opportunities. Assess student's mastery of the procedure within the specified situation.

CONSEQUENT EVENT REGULATION, ANTECEDENT CUE REGULATION, AND SELF-DETERMINATION

We now return to the role of these strategies within the consequent event regulation process to promote self-determination and self-determined learning. Table 7.1 depicts the relationship between antecedent cue and consequent event regulation and self- versus other-determined and directed behavior. The rows in the table classify antecedent event regulation as self- or other-controlled, and the columns in the table classify consequent event regulation as being persistent or occasional. The

TABLE 7.1. Relationship between Antecedent and Consequent Event Regulation and Self- versus Other-Determined and Directed Behavior

Antecedent event regulation	Consequent event regulation	
	Persistent behavior regulation	Occasional behavior regulation
Self-regulated choosing	Self-determined behavior	Self-directed behavior
Other-regulated choosing	Other-determined behavior	Other-directed behavior

cells formed by the two regulation patterns distinguish between self- and other-determined behavior in column 1 and between self- and other-directed behavior in column 2. They identify the types of behavior commonly exhibited when we persistently regulate our behavior in accordance with our choices or in accordance with other people's choices and when we occasionally regulate our behavior in accordance with our choices or in accordance with other people's choices.

When we persistently regulate our behavior to enact our own choices, we exhibit self-determined behavior (cell 1), but when we persistently regulate our behavior to enact choices made by other people, we exhibit other-determined behavior. When we occasionally regulate our behavior to enact our own choices, we exhibit self-directed behavior (cell 3), and when we occasionally regulate our behavior to enact other people's choices, we exhibit other-directed behavior (cell 4).

Of course, none of us exhibits a particular type of behavior all the time. More likely, we exhibit all types routinely without noticing, which is functional in that it allows us to adjust to social life, where complying with the wishes of others is often as adaptive as is being self-determined. Still, there are some people who rarely act in a self-determined manner and who can benefit from learning to do so in their daily pursuits.

Figure 7.1 illustrates the functions of each of the strategies described in this chapter and Chapter 6 with repeated choice-making, goal-setting, and planning strategies promoting the self-agency required for self-determination, and self-monitoring, self-evaluation, self-reinforcement, and self-adjustment strategies promoting the regulatory persistence that is required.

This review of research on self-regulation suggests that, with a few modifications, some of these strategies can be used to promote self-determination in children and youth with disabilities. To clarify what we have in mind, compare the diagrams in Figures 7.2 and 7.3. Like Figure 7.1, Figure 7.2 graphically depicts the self-regulated behavior described in past research with the self-determined behavior we have targeted here. The shaded area identifies the behavior being self-managed due to its being controlled by self-monitoring, self-evaluation, and self-reinforcement strategies. Note how they function together to increase correspondence between behavior and any plan determined by someone other than the self. The resulting behavior is other-determined simply in that the self is not involved in choosing the plan. The nonshaded areas for antecedent event regulation indicate that lack of influence over the behavior being managed. Now consider Figure 7.3,

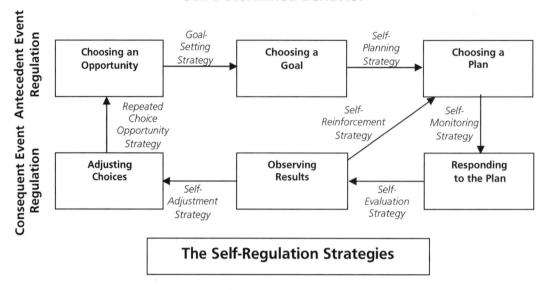

FIGURE 7.1. Strategies that affect antecedent and consequent event regulation during self-determination.

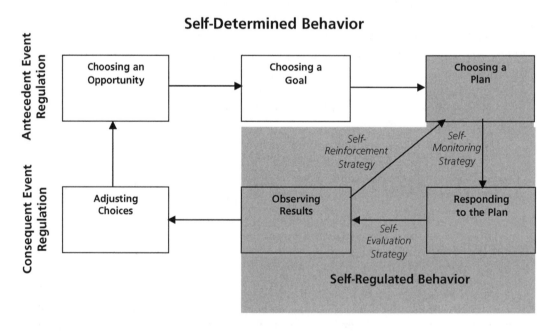

FIGURE 7.2. The relationship between self-determined and self-managed (self-directed) behavior.

Self-Determined Behavior

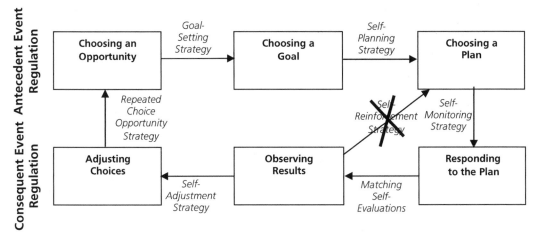

FIGURE 7.3. Matching during the regulation of self-determined behavior.

which shows how the choices of a person control the antecedents and how self-monitoring, self-evaluation, and self-adjustment (not self-reinforcement) strategies function to promote persistent responsiveness to those choices.

Some of our modifications to the use of self-regulation strategies are evident in Figure 7.3 as well. One of them is to focus the self-delivery of external rewards on matches between expectations and results in order to strengthen the relationship between goals set and results obtained. The purpose of this adjustment is to reinforce matches rather than compliance, correctness, or some other function unrelated to self-regulation. The second modification, as indicated in the figure, is to replace self-reinforcement with self-adjustment based on match results. This change produces adaptive effects in several ways. First, it motivates persistence in the pursuit of matches between goals and results. Second, it motivates repeated adjustments in choice and behavior until results match expectations. In other words, the self-determined pursuit eventually comes down to this pattern of persistent choosing, responding, comparing, and adjusting until there is a match.

Teaching the Regulation of Self-Determined Behavior

Our discussions of self-determined behavior and the strategies that promote it also have implications for teaching self-determination. One implication is that direct instruction is unlikely to be very effective because it requires teachers to control the antecedents and consequences that students must control in order to be self-determined. Another implication is that breaking self-determination into component elements in order to approximate successively a final skill set (self-determination) is, if the only approach, probably not as effective. Any deconstruction of the basic unit—choosing, responding to choice, adjusting, and choosing again—destroys the essential functions to be learned. Even deconstruction of choice making by teaching students there are good and bad choices is again a variation of teaching compliant behavior, in this case compliant verbal behavior. Standard instruction on use of behavior management strategies can lead down this path too, as indicated earlier in Figure 7.2.

From our perspective, the most promising option is also the simplest and most direct: teach students everything at once. We strongly recommend it because it puts the essential control functions in place for students to master as they choose and adjust to choice. Moreover, it is relatively easy to implement, even with immature learners who have yet to exhibit much self-determination. Consider the approach used with young children with severe disabilities illustrated in Figures 7.4 and 7.5. These children used a self-regulation card to learn all six self-regulation strategies at the same time. As indicated in the comment balloons of Figure 7.4, five strategies were located on the same card, and the sixth strategy—repeated choosing—was located across several cards used sequentially over time (Figure 7.5).

To learn antecedent and consequent strategy use, they completed the form, moving left to right, by choosing yes or no in columns 1–4. Then they totaled the number of yesses in the last row of column 4 and used that number to set goals for the number of matches they expected to achieve on the next card (see Figure 7.5). This is how they learned self-determination through matching. They learned to regulate the antecedents and consequences of their learning because they were allowed to use all six strategies repeatedly over time in order to get matches between what they expected (yes) and what they got (yes). This strategy let them learn about different choices, about choices that worked and choices that did not, as well as about choices that reflected what they liked and were capable of doing, essential knowledge for self-determination.

Last and perhaps most important, the teacher who implemented this approach reinforced matching rather than choosing or responding, which meant that her students learned to get yesses in their evaluation column, indicating that they accomplished what they claimed they would accomplish. They worked on the goal that they chose, and they completed work that their plan prescribed. The basis of success in any self-determined pursuit is achieving what one seeks to achieve, as opposed to other-determined pursuits, where achievement is in response to what others expect.

Were these young learners to continue to choose their goals and strive to produce results to meet them, they might develop into individuals who set one goal after another because of their success in previously met goals. Like these superachievers, they might become motivated less by extrinsic rewards associated with meeting a particular goal and more by the lure of meeting yet another, more challenging goal, as Brim (1992) explained:

> When we win, the response is to increase the degree of difficulty. We set a shorter timetable for the next endeavor, raising expectations for how much we can achieve, even broadening out and adding new goals. We will try to get there earlier or faster, and to get more or better.

1. By indicating Yes or No here, students **choose the goals** they want to meet for the upcoming autonomous work period.

2. By indicating Yes or No here, students **choose a plan** for meeting their goal in the upcoming autonomous work period.

3. By indicating Yes or No here, students **self-monitor** their behavior to determine whether they did what they planned to do.

4. By indicating Yes or No here, students used a **matching evaluation** to determine whether they met their goals.

Generic Self-Regulation Form			
Is My Goal Reading? Yes/No	**What Will I Do in Reading?** Read section in workbook Yes/No	**What Did I Do in Reading?** Read section in workbook Yes/No	**Did I Match (Meet) My Goal?** Yes/No
Is My Goal Math? Yes/No	**What Will I Do in Math?** Complete math worksheet Yes/No	**What Did I Do in Math?** Completed math worksheet Yes/No	**Did I Match (Meet) My Goal?** Yes/No
Is My Goal Science? Yes/No	**What Will I Do in Science?** Complete science worksheet Yes/No	**What Did I Do in Science?** Completed science worksheet Yes/No	**Did I Match (Meet) My Goal?** Yes/No
Is My Goal Social Studies? Yes/No	**What Will I Do in Social Studies?** Complete social studies worksheet Yes/No	**What Did I Do in Social Studies?** Completed social studies worksheet Yes/No	**Did I Match (Meet) My Goal?** Yes/No
Is My Goal Writing? Yes/No	**What Will I Do in Writing?** Write a journal entry Yes/No	**What Did I Do in Writing?** Wrote a journal entry Yes/No	**Did I Match (Meet) My Goal?** Yes/No
		Number of Goals Met (Yesses)?	
		Number of Goals Set (Yesses) *Next Time*?	

5. Difference between total Goals set this time, total Goals Met this time, and total Goals Set next time is **self-adjustment**.

FIGURE 7.4. How the self-regulation card helps learners master five strategies for self-determination.

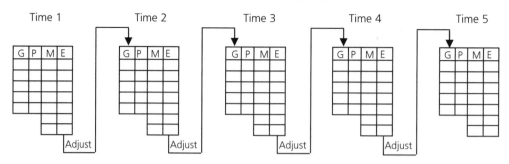

FIGURE 7.5. Use of multiple self-regulation cards to teach adjustments to repeated choice opportunities. G, goal-setting strategy; P, planning strategy; M, self-monitoring strategy; E, matching self-evaluation strategy; Adjust, self-adjustment strategy. Adapted from Mithaug, Martin, Agran, and Rusch (1988).

There are broad implications here for what happens to people when they are successful at work. Once you get good at a particular job, it no longer tasks most of your ability to do it well. So you set your sights higher and push on to more demanding work . . .

But there is a hitch. People can become psychologically trapped by their own success as they race to keep up with the rising expectations bred by each new achievement. With each success, they raise their level of difficulty, climbing the ladder of subgoals, moving faster, raising aspirations, and at some point reaching the limit of their capacity. (pp. 31–32)

SUMMARY

A common misconception about promoting self-determination is that it should commence with big choices—what you want to be when you grow up, what you want to do when you go to school, what you want to do today, what you want to learn. Although questions like these are provocative enough to engage students in interesting conversations, they are not necessary to develop competencies in the types of self-regulatory behavior covered here. On the contrary, small choice opportunities serve this purpose better, as illustrated in Figure 7.4. For that group of immature learners, a yes or no choice for subjects that were routinely required in daily classroom work constituted an occasion for learning to be self-determined.

Another misguided view is that teaching self-determination must wait until students are ready, until they are sufficiently self-controlled or self-regulated to benefit. Again, this is off the mark in that there are no prerequisites for learning to be self-determined, nor is there any ceding of ultimate control or authority to students who cannot control themselves. Look at the columns of the self-regulation card in Figure 7.4. A teacher selected that menu of options for a group of students who lacked self-control. Nonetheless, they were able to use the strategies embedded in the cards to exhibit self-determined behavior.

Finally, the endgame of this quest to promote self-determination is rarely discussed or considered in the literature, which would seem fully to justify advocating it for all students: to get students "hooked" on meeting their goals. Indeed, there is motivational magic in the self-determined pursuit, as most achievers can attest. Csikszentmihalyi (1990) found this in his research on the types of activities people find most enjoyable in their lives. He called the source of this enjoyment "flow":

> The optimal state of inner experience is one in which there is order in consciousness. This happens when psychic energy—or attention—is invested in realistic goals and when skills match the opportunities for action. The pursuit of a goal brings order in awareness because a person must concentrate attention on the task at hand and momentarily forget everything else. These periods of struggling to overcome challenge are what people find to be the most enjoyable times of their lives. . . . A person who has achieved control over psychic energy and has invested it in consciously chosen goals cannot help but grow into a more complex being. By stretching skills, by reaching toward higher challenges, such a person becomes an increasingly ordinary individual. (Csikszentmihalyi, 1990, p. 6)

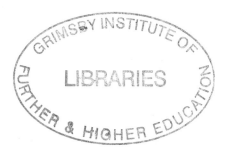

CHAPTER 8

Self-Instruction

Self-instruction involves students making task-specific statements out loud prior to or concurrent with their performance of a task. That is, they are taught to tell themselves what they need to do. These verbalizations serve as antecedents for the desired behavior. By having the verbalizations precede or accompany the desired behavior, it is hoped that the likelihood of that behavior being performed is increased.

Teaching students to self-instruct enables them to direct their own learning and performance of tasks and, as such, enables them to become more self-determined learners. Self-instruction is a verbal strategy students use with varying degrees of success and is of particular value for students with intellectual and developmental disabilities in the context of inclusive classrooms (Agran, King-Sears, Wehmeyer, & Copeland, 2003). It is, arguably, the most portable and adaptable educational support available.

Because many students with intellectual and developmental disabilities may have difficulty with short-term memory and problem solving, self-instruction provides a student with self-directed verbalizations to cue desired responses. Also, it allows a student verbally to rehearse what he or she needs to do and to engage in meaningful problem solving. Since our behavior is largely controlled by language, self-instruction allows students to direct their own behavior—a valued skill if someone is to become more self-determined.

Teaching self-instruction involves a two-step process: teaching the student (1) to repeat the self-instructions and (2) to complete the task at the same time or after each self-instruction is uttered. To ensure that the self-instruction serves a function, behavioral performance is monitored to identify a consistent "say–do correspondence." That is, it is observed if the verbalization consistently precedes or accompanies the execution of the desired behavior. When teaching self-instruction, the student's communicative capacity dictates the nature of the language employed. Consequently, self-instruction has been taught using verbal language, signing, and communication boards. What is most important is that the targeted words, signs, or pictures are produced prior to or at the same time as the performance of the desired response.

FUNCTIONAL EFFICACY OF SELF-INSTRUCTION

Several explanations of self-instruction have been suggested. First, self-instruction has been explained as an additional environmental cue or stimulus to increase the probability that a desired behavior will follow (Agran, 1997; Hughes & Lloyd, 1993; Malott, 1984). The self-instruction cues the behavior, which is followed by a consequence that reinforces the behavior (Hughes, 1997). Additionally, self-instruction may have a reinforcing property. In a self-instruction set (i.e., the verbalizations that make up a specific self-instruction strategy) the last verbalization may often include a verbal reinforcer or praise statement. For example, after repeating the task-related self-instructions and completing the task, the student is taught to say, "Great job! I finished all the math problems." This statement may in and of itself serve as the positive consequence for performance of the target behavior.

Second, since language and thought are integrally linked, self-instruction has also been advanced as a verbal mediator, which can regulate or control behavior (Whitman, 1990). Luria (1961) suggested that the internalization of speech provides the child a basis of self-regulation of behavior and increased control over the environment. Similarly, Vygotsky (1962) suggested that the ability of individuals to regulate their own behavior stems from the internalization of adult verbal regulations. Young children internalize the regulations and verbal information that adults provide. These verbalizations are transformed into private speech and essentially function as regulatory thought processes that allow the child to problem solve and regulate goal-directed behavior. Self-instruction functions similarly, serving as overt private speech that allows children to plan, organize, and regulate their own behavior. In this respect, self-instruction is thought of as mediating behavior and influences the way the student thinks about a behavioral event. Teaching students to self-instruct provides a self-directed instructional support for those students who do not utilize private speech.

The school, home, and community environments children participate in are largely language environments in which their behavior is controlled by the language of others (e.g., teachers, parents, siblings). Self-instruction allows children to control their own behavior using their own language. In this respect, self-instruction is a potentially powerful self-directed learning strategy owing to the pervasive nature of language as a control agent.

SELF-INSTRUCTION AS A PROBLEM-SOLVING STRATEGY

Functioning successfully in school requires the ability to determine multiple solutions to multiple problems (Agran & Hughes, 1997). From the challenges of academic and other instructional tasks to knowing how best to behave across myriad school, community, social, and family situations, students are constantly challenged to determine the most efficient (as well as socially acceptable) behaviors to meet the requirements of different situations.

In Chapter 3, we discussed strategies to promote problem solving. Feuerstein (1979, 1980) suggested that children with learning difficulties often have difficulty in problem solving because they lack mediated learning experiences. In their varied environmental interactions, children are exposed to many stimuli but are unable to transform them (i.e., develop learning sets)—transformation is done for them by others. As a result, many students with intellectual and developmental disabilities experience problems at one or more of the following levels: input (the reception of data), elaboration (the use of data), or output (communication or implementation of solution). By modifying cognitive processes or mediation, "individuals are able to frame, filter, and schedule direct stimuli themselves" (Feuerstein, 1980, p. 16).

The function of teaching students self-instruction strategies is so they can provide themselves with internal cues. Such cues, Senf (1976) suggested, can provide students with a feedback loop in which they can encode incoming information and provide it with relevance by relating it to previously stored information. Students with disabilities need mediated learning experiences in which they are taught a cadre of problem-solving or critical thinking skills. Self-instruction serves to mediate such learning experiences.

SELF-INSTRUCTION TRAINING SEQUENCE

Teachers may choose from several models of self-instruction when teaching students to guide their own behavior, as illustrated in this section.

Self-Instruction with Individuals with Limited Verbal Skills

Hughes (1992) taught four adults with mental retardation to verbalize statements like those in Table 8.1 while solving problems related to household tasks. These statements were designed to be short and simple in response to the participants' limited verbal skills. The self-instruction a student will use is contingent on the task the student needs to complete and the behaviors desired. Also, the student's language capacity and ease in verbal communication will determine both the number of words and the specific verbalizations taught. The intent of self-instruction is to provide the student with sufficient verbal information to guide his or her behavior. There is no minimum or maximum number of words in any given self-instruction

TABLE 8.1. Self-Instructional Statements Related to Household Tasks

1. Identifying the problem (e.g., "not plugged in").
2. Stating the correct response (e.g., "got to plug in").
3. Evaluating the response (e.g., "fixed it").
4. Self-reinforcing (e.g., "good").

verbal set. For an individual who has restricted expressive language capacity, a short instruction (e.g., "I need help") may be sufficient. For a student involved in a multistep math division task, the number of verbalizations may be several. There are a number of self-instruction formats that have been investigated in the literature pertaining to students with intellectual and developmental disabilities.

Self-Instruction as a Problem-Solving Technique

Agran and Hughes (1997) suggested that self-instruction functions as a problem-solving strategy because it provides the student with relevant verbal cues to identify a problem, examine his or her skill repertoire for effective responses previously used in the same or a similar situation, direct him- or herself to perform that action, and evaluate the action taken. Self-instruction in effect provides the student with a self-regulated learning strategy. An example of a problem-solving self-instruction is presented in Table 8.2.

Self-Instruction as a Task-Sequencing Strategy

Students with intellectual and developmental disabilities may have difficulty completing complex task sequences (e.g., setting up a chemical experiment). A self-instruction strategy found useful in facilitating task completion is the Did–Next–Now approach (Agran & Moore, 1994). In this strategy, the student learns to perform the first response in the sequence, then verbally state what he or she has just performed ("Did"). The student states what he or she needs to do next ("Next"), then verbally directs him- or herself to perform this response ("Now"). This verbal set is performed for each response in the sequence.

Did–Next–Now is especially useful for teaching students to perform a series of tasks in a sequence (e.g., loading a commercial dishwasher, writing an essay). A

TABLE 8.2. Problem-Solving Self-Instruction

1. Identifying the problem (e.g., "I want to talk").
2. Stating the correct response (e.g., "I need to look and talk").
3. Evaluating the response (e.g., "I did it. I talked").
4. Self-reinforcing (e.g., "I did a good job").

strategy script for designing a Did–Next–Now self-instruction program is provided in Figure 8.1. The script prompts the teacher to identify a preceding response (e.g., sweeping the floor), a Did–Next–Now verbal sequence (e.g., "I swept the floor. I have to empty the trash. I need to do it now"), a subsequent target response (e.g., emptying the trash), a reinforcer to follow and maintain the target response ("Good job. Look at that floor"), and a correction procedure to use in case of error (e.g., "Oops. I was supposed to empty the trash next. Guess I better do that now"). Using this strategy, Agran, Fodor-Davis, and Moore (1986) taught job-sequencing skills to four students with mental retardation enrolled in a hospital work skills program. The students stated the Did–Next–Now verbal sequence when performing a 21-step task sequence for cleaning patient rooms, which included tasks such as dusting and cleaning restrooms. The sequence was repeated each time the students began a new step of the sequence (e.g., "I just brought the bucket to the room. I need to fill the bucket. I'm going to fill the bucket now").

Self-Instruction as a Direction-Following Strategy

Because students with intellectual disabilities may have difficulty understanding what is expected of them, following directions may be very problematic. The What/Where strategy is designed to provide students with a strategy in which they can produce additional cues that inform them what they are supposed to do and where they are supposed to do it. Students are taught to select key words from an oral or written instruction and to determine *what* they are to do and *where* to do it. For example, a student may be told by the teacher, "These are the stencils. They go on the back table." Using the What/Where strategy, the student would repeat, "Stencils. Back table," while beginning to put the stencils away. Figure 8.2 is an example of this strategy.

Self-Instruction as an Interactive Strategy

By function, self-instruction involves "talking-out" behavior. That is, students provide to themselves verbal cues that would otherwise be provided by another person. As a self-directed instructional strategy, self-instruction allows students to produce additional verbal information that may greatly enhance their autonomy and self-determination and, in effect, provide their own support; however, it is evident that talking aloud is typically not considered socially appropriate and may further marginalize the student. To address this issue, the Did–Next–Ask strategy within the interactive self-instruction model, provides a socially acceptable self-instruction within the context of a social interaction.

The interactive self-instruction model teaches students to state their self-instructions as questions embedded in conversation. This strategy is particularly useful when a student is interacting with others in public, and self-instructing aloud would draw attention to him or her. Rather than emitting self-instruction in a directive format (e.g., "Go the next number"), the student instead provides the self-

Student: _____ Setting: _____

Instructional Target: _____ Task: _____

Preceding Response	Verbalization (what student says)	Target Response (what student should do)	Reinforcer	Correction Procedure
	Did: Next: Now:			
	Did: Next: Now:			
	Did: Next: Now:			
	Did: Next: Now:			

FIGURE 8.1. Did–Next–Now self-instruction strategy.

Student: _____ Setting: _____

Instructional Target: _____ Task: _____

Target Response (what student should do)	Antecedent Stimuli	Verbalization (What student says)	Reinforcer	Correction Procedure
	What: Where:			
	What: Where:			
	What: Where:			
	What: Where:			

FIGURE 8.2. What/Where self-instruction strategy.

instruction in the form of a question (e.g., "What is the next number?") In the present context, the Did–Next–Ask strategy is used in a social interaction in which the student is taught to repeat in the form of a question a verbalization that he or she has just heard. This is a rhetorical strategy that many people use to ensure they correctly heard what someone said (e.g., "Did you say that . . .?") and is suggested for situations in which more directive verbalizations may be devaluing to the speaker. This strategy is particularly suitable for those situations in which the student is providing a service to the teacher or other students (e.g., obtaining materials). Similar to the Did–Next–Now strategy, the interactive model involves teaching the student to remind him- or herself of the task step just completed. The second verbalization reminds the student what he or she needs to do next. The last verbalization involves a question about the next step in the sequence. Figure 8.3 is an example of this strategy.

ADVANTAGES OF SELF-INSTRUCTION

One advantage of self-instruction for promoting learning in general education settings is its adaptability. Self-instruction can be used to teach a wide variety of academic and social skills (e.g., initiating conversations, following directions). Unlike other student-directed strategies (e.g., picture or audio prompt systems), self-instruction does not require that students carry materials with them as they perform activities. Once students have learned the sequence of statements or questions they will use to guide their behavior, they can begin to verbalize these prompts silently or using a whisper.

Self-Instruction to Promote Generalization

Being able to apply or transfer skills learned in one setting or with one individual to a new setting or person is an important goal for *all* students. Many students with intellectual and developmental disabilities don't achieve this outcome unless they receive instruction that specifically teaches generalization of an acquired skill. "Generalization" of behavior is demonstrated when students perform targeted skills in situations not associated with instruction (i.e., when they encounter unique situations, people, tasks, or demands) and when their performance continues over time following withdrawal of instruction (i.e., maintenance) (Berg, Wacker, & Flynn, 1990; Pierce & Schreibman, 1994). Although the importance of generalization as a educational goal is widely accepted, strategies to promote generalization are rarely incorporated into instructional programs (Bandura, 1969; Shore, Iwata, Lerman, & Shirley, 1994; Stokes & Baer, 1977). To promote generalization, teachers typically provide cues across different settings so that students have the opportunity to practice a given skill in these settings, but if the teacher is not available, the student may not be sufficiently cued to perform the desired response. Self-instruction provides a potentially powerful means to promote generalization

Student: _____ Setting: _____

Instructional Target: _____ Task: _____

Preceding Response	Verbalization (what student says)	Target Response (what student should do)	Reinforcer	Correction Procedure
	Did: Next: Ask:			
	Did: Next: Ask:			
	Did: Next: Ask:			
	Did: Next: Ask:			

FIGURE 8.3. Interactive self-instruction strategy.

because it allows the student to produce the appropriate cue whenever and however often it may be needed. Specific recommendations for promoting generalization when teaching students to self-instruct are described later in this chapter.

EVIDENCE-BASED RESEARCH FOR SELF-INSTRUCTION

Self-instruction has been investigated for approximately the last four decades, and a variety of research methodologies have been employed to investigate the effects of self-instruction on diverse learning and adaptive skills. For example, Guralnick (1976) investigated the effects of self-instruction training on the matching-to-sample skills of 32 children with intellectual disabilities. The children were randomly assigned to one of four groups: self-instruction training, modeling-only, feedback-only, and control. The training for the self-instruction group consisted of modeling verbalizations and corresponding motor behavior, then fading from audible to covert self-instruction. In addition, the self-instruction group was provided with a problem-solving strategy that involved training the children to be familiar with a sample of forms, to differentiate the critical dimensions of the stimuli, and to eliminate incorrect alternatives by checking with a standard. The modeling-only group observed the same modeling of verbalizations and behavior as the self-instruction group but did not receive self-instruction training. The feedback-only group did not receive modeling or self-instruction training but received feedback on performance. Guralnick reported a statistically significant difference between the self-instruction group and the other three groups on the posttest assessment, which suggested that the self-instruction training best facilitated the acquisition of the target behavior.

This section of the chapter presents an overview of current empirical studies in which self-instruction strategies have been taught to people with intellectual and developmental disabilities in school, work, and residential environments. Studies are grouped according to content or skill areas specific to each environment.

Teaching Self-Instruction in School Environments

Academic Skills

Whitman and colleagues investigated the effects of self-instruction on mathematics performance for students with intellectual disabilities in a series of studies. Johnston, Whitman, and Johnson (1980) and Whitman and Johnston (1983) taught students with mild intellectual disabilities to add and subtract numbers with regrouping. The self-instruction involved a series of questions based on a task analysis of the computational process. When students were taught to self-instruct, increases were reported in accuracy of problems completed, but rate of completion decreased. The authors speculated that, over time, self-instruction might require less effort by students and, subsequently, rate of performance would increase.

Using the same self-instruction format, Keogh, Whitman, and Maxwell (1988) compared the effects of self-instruction and teacher-delivered instruction on rate and accuracy of adding with regrouping by students with and without mild intellectual disabilities. Students without disabilities improved their accuracy following both instructional conditions and their rate following teacher-delivered instruction only. Only the self-instruction condition resulted in improvements in rate and accuracy for students with intellectual disabilities.

Agran and colleagues (Agran, Cavin, Wehmeyer, & Palmer, 2006) studied the effects of self-instruction training in promoting inclusive practice and access to the general education curriculum for students with intellectual and developmental disabilities. In one study, three students with intellectual disabilities were taught to self-regulate learning to achieve target goals—specifically, academic skills aligned with the district general curriculum standards (Agran et al., 2006). Students were responsible for choosing both the target behavior and the student-directed learning strategy. The target behaviors across students included: practicing methods of scientific inquiry, understanding different types of maps, and learning about the organ systems of the body. Two of the students selected self-instruction as the instructional strategy to achieve self-selected goals. One student who was interested in learning how to read maps and his teacher developed an invented sign language that corresponded to each step of a self-monitoring and self-instruction procedure (for example, "What type of information am I looking for?"; "What types of maps do I have to choose from?"; "Which one would work best?"; and "Pick it"). For the second student, self-instruction served as an augmentative learning strategy and involved the verbalizations "look, point, match." The teacher demonstrated the strategy by giving a cue ("Where is the nervous system, and what does it do?"), followed by stating "look" (while looking at the choices), then "point" (pointing at the correct choice), and "match" (while matching the picture cue of the system with its function). Both students achieved the mastery criterion level (i.e., 80% correct responding across three consecutive sessions).

In a second study, two out of three junior high school students with intellectual and developmental disabilities in a family consumer class were taught to use self-instruction to improve their skills in asking for assistance in class and cooking, respectively (Agran et al., 2005). Both students achieved the mastery criterion of 80% correct responding.

Community Living and Work Skills

Wacker and colleagues (Wacker, Carroll, & Moe, 1980; Wacker & Greenebaum, 1984) taught sorting and assembly skills to students with intellectual disabilities. Their abbreviated self-instruction method required that students say aloud only the color or shape of cards as they sorted or assembled the cards in sequence. The teacher demonstrated the correct performance of the required task sequence while stating aloud the color or shape of the cards being sorted or assembled. During subsequent instructional sessions, the students were taught to say the names of the colors or shapes without prompting while independently completing the assembly steps. Students in both studies improved their accuracy on required tasks following training and generalized their skills from the instructional setting to the regular classroom. In addition, using a group-comparison design, Wacker and Greenebaum (1984) demonstrated that self-instruction was more effective than direct instruction at producing task acquisition and that only self-instruction produced generalization across related responses.

Hughes, Hugo, and Blatt (1996) taught a domestic skill (i.e., making toast) to five high school students with severe intellectual disabilities. The toast-making sequence was divided into 10 tasks. Five problem-solving tasks were used as training examples (i.e., multiple exemplars), and the remaining five served as generalization probes. First, students were taught to self-instruct in response to one of the five training examples. When students were proficient at self-instructing with one example, the remaining four training examples were introduced. All five students learned to self-instruct while performing the training tasks and to generalize their use of the strategy to the untrained tasks, performing all steps of the toast-making task in sequence. In addition, performance across both trained and untrained tasks was maintained after instructional support was withdrawn.

Social and Interpersonal Skills

Collet-Klingenberg and Chadsey-Rusch (1991) taught three high school students in vocational training with intellectual disabilities to respond appropriately to constructive criticism. The students were taught to verbalize four different types of statements ("decoding," "decision-making," "performing," and "self-evaluating") in response to five hand-drawn pictures depicting social situations in which employees were receiving work-related criticism from their supervisors. The statements were role-played by the students and a trainer in response to the scenarios indicated in the pictures. Findings indicated that two of the students learned to perform the cognitive process and to generalize appropriate responding to new role-play scenes involving criticism. No generalization was observed for the student who did not acquire the cognitive process, indicating that this adaptation of the self-instruction process may have been critical to the generalization of social skills.

Hughes, Harmer, Killian, and Niarhos (1995) taught four high school students with intellectual disabilities to initiate and respond to conversation with a variety of familiar and unfamiliar peers with and without disabilities. Peers without disabilities taught the students to self-instruct during conversation skills training. In addition, the peers modeled interactive conversation characteristic of typical high school students and provided corrective feedback and reinforcement to the students as they learned their new conversation skills. Following self-instruction training by peers, all four students learned to initiate and maintain conversation with new partners in a variety of high school settings. In addition, the students' conversation skills compared favorably to those of a group of typical high school students without disabilities. Hughes and colleagues (2000) used self-instruction in combination with a communication booklet to teach high school students with intellectual disabilities to increase their social interaction with their general education peers. Peer "buddies" taught the students to use their self-instructions to engage in interactive conversations with their general education classmates and to use their conversation booklets to ask questions of their conversation partners.

Teaching Self-Instruction in Work Environments

Teaching self-instruction skills has been extended to settings in which people with intellectual and developmental disabilities are employed. Areas of focus include (1) work skills, (2) productivity, (3) academic skills, and (4) social and interpersonal skills.

Work Skills

Wacker and colleagues (1988) adapted the self-instruction strategy used in school settings (e.g., Wacker et al., 1980) for students with intellectual disabilities who were receiving vocational evaluations in a university-based work setting. When entering data into a computer, calculator, or checkbook, the students were taught to self-instruct each letter, number, or character as it was entered. Following self-instruction training, all students increased their accuracy of data entry across trained and untrained data entry tasks. In addition, when asked if they found self-instruction disruptive, the students' coworkers responded that they were not aware that the students were talking aloud.

Agran, Fodor-Davis, Moore, and Deer (1989) used a What/Where self-instruction strategy script to teach instruction-following skills to five students with intellectual disabilities enrolled in a janitorial program. The students were taught to say to themselves what they were supposed to do and where they were supposed to do it after they were given an instruction. For example, the students were taught to say "Vacuum under table" when they were told to vacuum the carpet under the table or "Wipe front stove" when given an instruction to wipe the front of a stove. All students were found to improve their instruction-following skills across trained and untrained situations when they used their self-instructions.

Hughes and Rusch (1989) combined self-instruction with multiple exemplars of targeted responses to teach two workers with severe intellectual and developmental disabilities employed at a soap-packaging company to solve work-related problems. First, the work supervisor identified problem situations that were likely to occur during the workday, such as a puddle of soap on a table where work was to be completed or a paper towel plugging the drain of a sink. Next, the employees were taught to self-instruct in response to five of the identified problem situations.

Acquisition of the problem-solving strategy was demonstrated in addition to generalized application of the strategy to untrained problem situations.

Productivity

An adaptation of self-instruction called "verbal correspondence" was used by Crouch, Rusch, and Karlan (1984) to improve kitchen workers' start times, productivity, and supervisor ratings when performing kitchen tasks, such as sweeping, mopping, and setting up food on a lunch line. Using this procedure, the employees were taught to say the times at which they would start and complete their work. First, they were reinforced for stating the correct times. Next, they were reinforced each time their stated times and actual start and completion times were the same. Stating their start and completion times increased the rate of production of all employees and improved their supervisors' ratings of their performance.

Rusch, Martin, Lagomarcino, and White (1987) used an adaptation of self-instruction correspondence called "verbal mediation" to teach a woman with an intellectual disability employed in a fast-food restaurant to state her required job sequences (i.e., 23 set-up and clean-up tasks) before performing those tasks. Tasks included clearing tables, taking out trash, wiping tables and counters, and sweeping and mopping the dining area. The verbal mediation strategy required the employee to state in detail each step of the job sequence before performing the required responses. Using verbal mediation, she learned to perform tasks in sequence as well as to generalize her skills across scheduled changes in task demands.

Moore, Agran, and Fodor-Davis (1989) examined the effects of a self-management program involving self-instruction, goal setting, and self-reinforcement on the productivity of four employees with severe intellectual disabilities employed in a sheltered workshop. The participants were responsible for a packaging task. They were instructed to set performance goals for themselves, to tell themselves to work faster, and to reinforce themselves with coins when they met their criteria. After training, all participants increased and maintained their production rates at criterion levels for up to 3 months.

Academic Skills

Browder and Minarovic (2000) taught three adults with intellectual disabilities employed in competitive employment a variety of sight words relevant to their jobs. A two-part instructional program was employed. First, the participants were shown flash cards on which the words were printed. Second, a Did–Next–Now strategy was used in which the participants were taught to use the sight words to indicate which step in the work task they had just completed and which they needed to do next, then to direct themselves to complete that step. All participants achieved mastery levels for the target behavior.

Social and Interpersonal Skills

Adaptations of self-instruction procedures have been applied to teach employees with intellectual and developmental disabilities to seek assistance when needed to complete tasks. Agran, Salzberg, and Stowitschek (1987) taught five employees in a vocational training setting to initiate requests when they were out of materials or in need of assistance. The employees were taught to self-instruct the problem and the response when they needed help to complete tasks involved with unpacking cheese, assembling recliner chairs and irrigation wheels, and making candles. For example, employees would say to themselves "I am out of _____" (stating the problem) and "I need to get more _____. I'll ask for _____" (stating the response). Next, the employees would ask a supervisor for assistance. After self-instruction training, participants increased their requests for assistance in both the training and work setting.

Using a teaching format similar to that reported in Agran and colleagues (1987), Rusch, McKee, Chadsey-Rusch, and Renzaglia (1988) taught a young man with a severe intellectual and physcal disabilities employed in a university-operated film center to make appropriate requests when (1) materials were not available or (2) materials ran out. The employee's job was to receive, fill, and deliver orders for desk supplies to clerical workers. When materials were unavailable or ran out, the young man was taught to state "Can't [complete order]." He then would tap a picture of a teacher's aide that was taped to his wheelchair, and say "Tell [the aide]." Next, he was taught to approach the aide, establish eye contact, say "Excuse me," and request the missing items by saying "I need more [name of item]." Following completion of all self-instruction steps, the employee was taught to reinforce himself with a nickel. His requests for assistance increased when the young man performed his self-instruction steps.

Rusch, Morgan, Martin, Riva, and Agran (1985) and Hughes and Petersen (1989) taught employees with mild to moderate intellectual disabilities to increase their time on task while performing required job-related tasks. Employees in these studies were taught to ask, "What does [the supervisor] want me to do?" (stating the problem), then say "I am supposed to wipe the counter and restock the supplies" (stating the response), "OK, I wiped the counter" (self-evaluating), and "Good. I did that right" (self-reinforcing). To prompt self-instruction, Hughes and Petersen placed on the employees' work tables photographs that showed the employees busy working. Following self-instruction training, increases in time spent working generalized from the training to the work situation for employees across both studies.

Teaching Self-Instruction in Community Living and Recreational Environments

Hughes (1992) taught four residents of a group home who had severe intellectual disabilities to solve task-related problems. Four problem situations served as training tasks (i.e., multiple exemplars), and four served as generalization probes. The combined strategy was associated with generalization to untrained problems for all residents, as well as maintenance of the problem-solving strategy (i.e., responding to multiple exemplars and self-instructing).

Keogh, Faw, Whitman, and Reid (1984) used self-instruction to teach two adolescent boys with behavior problems who lived in a community residence to play board games. The boys were taught to state the correct response by verbalizing individual game steps as they played. Both boys increased performance and verbalization of game steps when instruction was introduced sequentially across games. Prompts and additional instruction were required before generalization occurred in dyad and free-play situations; generalization to three untrained games did not occur. Game skills were maintained, although occasional instructional sessions were required.

Summary of Empirical Studies

As indicated in the above review, investigations of the effects of self-instruction on persons with intellectual and developmental disabilities have been conducted across school, work, and residential settings. Self-instruction was found to be effective at increasing proficiency in the areas of academic skills, daily living skills, social skills, productivity, and employment skills. Self-instruction was also found to be effective in producing generalization and maintenance of target behaviors to varying degrees across studies.

INSTRUCTIONAL RECOMMENDATIONS

Teaching self-instruction is relatively straightforward and cost-effective. Several researchers have suggested that instruction takes approximately 2 hours, either in one session or in 30-minute sessions across 4 to 5 days. (Note: For students with more significant support needs, additional time may be required.) Additionally, self-instruction training can be taught using an individual or group format. When the self-instructions are similar for all students, group instruction is strongly recommended, as it provides more practice time for all members of the group. Further, there is a growing body of research suggesting that peer tutors, both with and without disabilities, can teach other students to self-instruct (Agran & Moore, 1994; Hughes et al., 1996, 2000). The advantage of using peer tutors is twofold: it can reduce teacher instructional time, and it can be highly motivating to students receiving instruction. Peer tutors deliver the instructional program the same way as teachers, following the task analysis and instructional sequence of the program. Reinforcement and feedback to the peer tutors are provided as necessary. Role plays provide an appropriate context for instruction.

Typically, self-instruction comprises complete phrases or sentences. These phrases need to contain sufficient information for the student to attend to the salient dimensions of the task. For students who have communication disorders, it may be necessary to shorten the self-instruction and use only a word or two. For example, if the student has difficulty saying, "I need to write between the lines," it may be necessary to teach him or her to say only, "write between lines."

Additionally, for students who have difficulty learning to self-instruct, other educational supports may be taught concurrently. If task completion can be enhanced by teaching the student to self-instruct and refer to picture cues or to reinforce him- or herself, those supports may be appropriate. Again, the focus of self-instruction is to get the student to attend to task requirements. Additional support strategies may serve as additional cues for desired responding or as more immediate and powerful reinforcers.

The following instructional sequence is recommended for teaching self-instruction (Agran et al., 2003).

Step 1: Provide Rationale

The first step in the process is to provide a rationale to the student for the value of self-instruction. The teacher must make an effort to inform the student about the appropriateness of the strategy for the target behavior. Target behavior selection should be based on the student's wishes, preferences, and self-determined needs, with input from parents, teachers, and related personnel or peers. Based on this selection, specified student-directed strategies (e.g., self-instruction, self-monitoring) are suggested based on demonstrated effectiveness, ease of use, and, of course, the student's preferences.

Students who are aware of negative social consequences of talking aloud may be reluctant to select self-instruction as a strategy or consistently use it. If a student has a concern about the strategy's social acceptance but is willing to use it, he or she may be told to self-instruct quietly so as not to get negative attention.

Step 2: Teacher Models and Self-Instructs

For this step, the teacher models the behavior and self-instructions, and the student observes. After the self-instructions have been designed specific to the task, the teacher models the self-instructions and the behaviors required to complete the task. The student is instructed to listen to what the teacher says and does. In particular, the student is reminded that self-instruction precedes the response.

Step 3: Teacher Instructs and Student Performs

As in Step 2, this step also involves task completion and self-instruction, but this time the teacher self-instructs and the student engages in the task either after the instruction or at the same time. Performing the task and self-instructing at the same time may initially be too difficult for students, hence the need for phasing in self-instruction. The student is instructed to pay attention to the self-instruction and is given feedback on his or her task performance.

Step 4: Student Performs and Instructs

In this step, the student is asked to repeat the self-instructions and to perform the target behavior either after or at the same time as the self-instructions. After observing the teacher demonstrate both the self-instructions and task performance, the student can now perform all of these responses in contiguity. Prompting, reinforcement, and feedback are provided as needed. Although students may find concurrent self-instruction and task performance difficult, systematic instruction and positive feedback will remind the student of the correspondence between the two; that is, execution of both will lead to task completion, which, in turn, will be reinforced. The need for consistent, systematic direct instructional methods in teaching students to self-instruct cannot be emphasized enough (Hughes, 1997). In addition to learning the responses needed to complete the task, self-instruction also necessitates that the student emit a set of verbalizations. As stated previously, this aspect may be challenging for many students. Consequently, instruction needs to be as precise and reinforcing as possible to ensure successful outcomes—completion of the task and consistent utterance of the self-instructions to ensure the former.

Step 5: Student Performs and Instructs Covertly

The last step in teaching self-instruction is to ensure that the student internalizes the self-instructions. First, request that the student whisper the self-instructions after he or she has demonstrated being able to repeat them aloud. Next, teach the student to self-instruct so that the self-instructions cannot be heard. As stated earlier in this chapter, it is believed that, once internalized, specific self-instructions will function to mediate or guide behavior, but as mentioned previously, it should be noted that many recent self-instruction applications do not include this step (see Hughes, 1997). In the case of self-instruction, it is hoped that a say–do relationship has been established; that is, did the student consistently self-instruct prior to or at the same time as each step in the task? Is the student indeed self-instructing—either audibly or through lip movements? As a compromise, Hughes (1997) recommended that teachers may request that their students self-instruct aloud when they are present but refrain from overtly self-instructing when in the company of others. This potential problem may also be resolved by asking key stakeholders (the student, peers, staff) their opinions on the appropriateness of spoken self-instructions in public situations. If these individuals find a student's self-instruction disruptive or objectionable, then teaching the student covert self-instruction is necessary. If the self-instruction is not objectionable, overt self-instruction is in order. In any case, students should be taught to self-instruct in as unobtrusive manner as possible.

Promoting Generalization

To promote generalized responding, the following instructional procedures are rec-ommended:

- Provide a number of examples of the type of task(s) you want students to learn. Be sure to provide self-instruction training across several different settings. For example, to teach students to use the Internet, you might choose to teach students self-instruction in the steps needed to access the Internet on the classroom computer and on computers in the school library. By varying the task slightly (computers in the two settings are not exactly the same) and providing instruction in different settings (the classroom and the library), it is more likely that students will successfully use their new skill in a new setting (for example, when in the school's technology lab or working on a computer at home).

- Include the same or similar cues in each different teaching setting. Including similar cues across different instructional settings is called "programming common stimuli." This teaching strategy helps students see the connections among using self-instruction in different situations, increasing the likelihood they will self-instruct across a range of situations.

- Finally, give students frequent reminders to self-instruct as they go through the day. This will result in frequent opportunities for students to practice their self-instruction strategies in many different settings and to perform tasks with less reliance on you or other adults. Most important, if appropriate, praise their use of self-instruction. Students will continue to self-instruct only if they realize that their self-instruction will consistently produce a desired outcome.

SUMMARY

Students and adults with intellectual and developmental disabilities have been taught self-instruction to address a wide range of academic, social, and community living and work skills. Self-instruction allows students to use their verbal behavior to guide their performance (Wehmeyer, Agran, & Hughes, 1998). Although the number of self-instruction studies involving students with intellectual and developmental disabilities remains limited (particularly in school settings), the studies do support the feasibility of teaching students with disabilities to use self-instruction to acquire, maintain, and generalize skills across a variety of tasks and conditions.

It is clear that, despite a growing body of evidence-based research to demonstrate the positive effects of self-instruction, relatively few people with severe intellectual and developmental disabilities are being taught to use this strategy (Brown, Gothelf, Guess, & Lehr, 1998; Powers, 2005). At one time it was believed that individuals with severe intellectual disabilities could not benefit from self-instruction training (Agran, 1997). As evidenced by the research on the effects of self-instruction, this contention has been invalidated. Nevertheless, because of the communicative challenges of people with intellectual and developmental disabilities, many educators and service providers may not believe that individuals with significant disabilities can benefit from self-instruction training. This misconception is indeed unfortunate, as self-instruction may serve as a useful means for individuals to cue and direct their own behavior when other supports are not available. As mentioned previously, self-instruction is the most portable self-directed learning strategy and has wide applicability to a variety of learning and adaptive situations. Verbal self-regulation and rehearsal is a strategy typical students use to varying degrees and may be a very powerful means to promote self-determination.

CHAPTER 9

The Self-Determined Learning Model of Instruction

In Chapter 1 of this book, we emphasized that self-determination develops as young people become more capable of or are provided supports to make choices and express preferences, set and attain goals, recognize and solve problems, participate in and make decisions, and self-regulate their behavior. Most of the intervening chapters have provided information on strategies to enable teachers to teach students the skills they need to attain these component elements.

Like with many instructional efforts, it is often more powerful to combine strategies into a multicomponent model. Further, as we discussed in Chapter 7, for students to self-determine learning, they need to have the opportunity to be causal agents in the learning process. Over the past decade, we have been engaged in the development and validation of a model of teaching that provides a framework within which to implement such a multicomponent intervention to promote self-determination and student-directed learning. This instructional model, the self-determined learning model of instruction (SDLMI), is described in this chapter.

Joyce and Weil (1980) defined a model of teaching as "a plan or pattern that can be used to shape curriculums (long term courses of study), to design instructional materials, and to guide instruction in the classroom and other settings" (p. 1). Such models are derived from theories about human behavior, learning, or cognition, and effective teachers employ multiple models of teaching, taking into account the unique characteristics of the learner and type of learning.

Like all educators, teachers working with students with intellectual and developmental disabilities use a variety of teaching models, based on a student's learning characteristics and the content under consideration. A teacher may use the role-playing model to teach social behaviors, social simulation and social inquiry models to examine social problems and solutions, assertiveness training to teach self-advocacy skills, or a training model to teach vocational skills. Likewise, special educators employ more traditional, cognitively-based models of teaching, such as the concept attainment model to teach thinking skills, the memory model for increasing the retention of facts, or the inductive thinking and inquiry training models to teach reasoning and academic skills. The teaching model most frequently adopted by special educators is the contingency management model, drawing on principles of operant psychology.

The common theme across these models of teaching is that they are teacher-directed. While they provide direction for strategy and curriculum development activities that can teach components of self-determination, none adequately provides teachers a model to enable young people truly to become causal agents in their own lives. The SDLMI (Mithaug, Wehmeyer, Agran, Martin, & Palmer, 1998) was developed to address this problem and is based on the component elements of self-determination, the process of self-regulated problem solving, and research on student-directed learning. It is appropriate for use with students with and without disabilities across a wide range of content areas and enables teachers to engage students in the totality of their educational programs by increasing opportunities to self-direct learning.

IMPLEMENTING THE MODEL

Implementation of the model consists of a three-phase instructional process depicted in Figures 9.1, 9.2, and 9.3. Each instructional phase presents a problem to be solved by the student. The student solves each problem by posing and answering a series of four student questions per phase that students learn, modify to make their own, and apply to reach self-selected goals. Each question is linked to a set of teacher objectives, and each instructional phase includes a list of educational supports that teachers can use to enable students to self-direct learning. In each instructional phase, the student is the primary agent for choices, decisions, and actions, even when eventual actions are teacher-directed.

STUDENT QUESTIONS

The student questions in the model are constructed to direct the student through a problem-solving sequence in each instructional phase. The solutions to the problems in each phase lead to the problem-solving sequence in the next phase. The construction of these questions was based on theory in the problem-solving and self-regulation literature that suggests there is a sequence of thoughts and actions, a means–ends problem-solving sequence, that must be followed for any person's actions to produce results that satisfy his or her needs and interests. Teachers

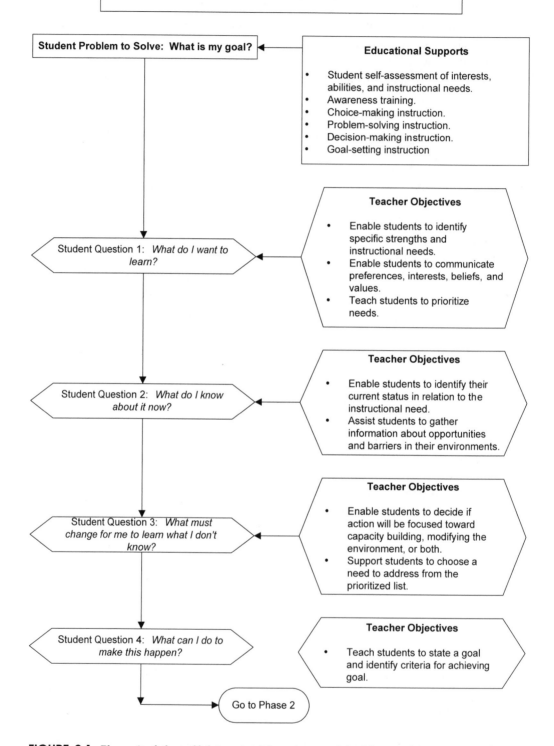

FIGURE 9.1. Phase 1 of the self-determined learning model of instruction. From Wehmeyer, Agran, and Hughes (1998). Copyright 1998 by Michael Wehmeyer, Martin Agran, and Carolyn Hughes. Reprinted by permission.

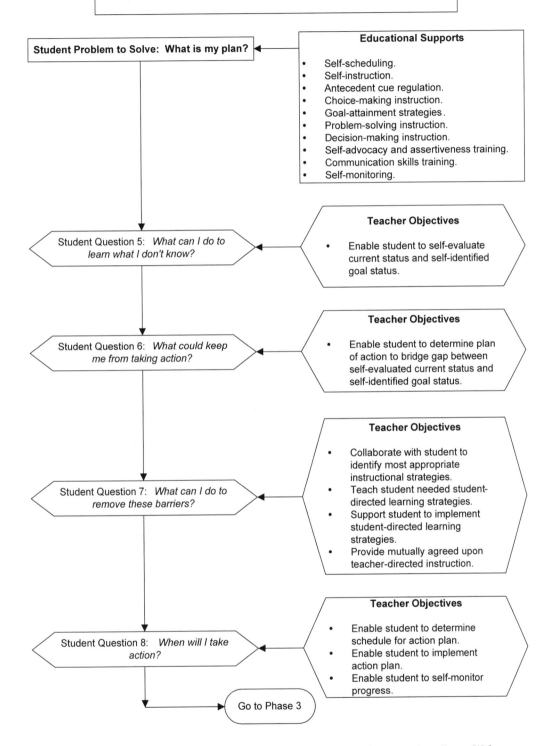

FIGURE 9.2. Phase 2 of the self-determined learning model of instruction. From Wehmeyer, Agran, and Hughes (1998). Copyright 1998 by Michael Wehmeyer, Martin Agran, and Carolyn Hughes. Reprinted by permission.

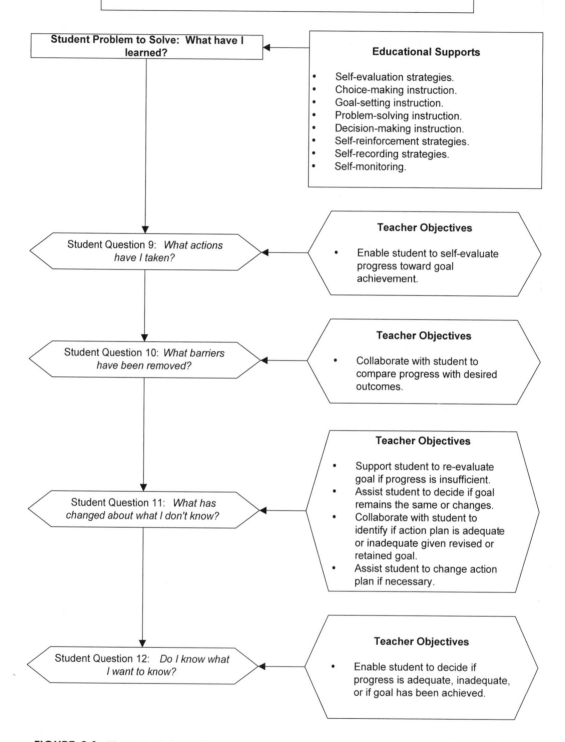

FIGURE 9.3. Phase 3 of the self-determined learning model of instruction. From Wehmeyer, Agran, and Hughes (1998). Copyright 1998 by Michael Wehmeyer, Martin Agran, and Carolyn Hughes. Reprinted by permission.

implementing the model teach students to solve a sequence of problems to construct a means–ends chain—a causal sequence—that moves them from where they are (an actual state of not having their needs and interests satisfied) to where they want to be (a goal state of having those needs and interests satisfied). Its function is to reduce or eliminate the discrepancy between what students want or need and what students currently have or know. The model constructs this means–ends sequence by having students answer the questions that connect their needs and interests to their actions and results via goals and plans.

To answer the questions in this sequence, students must regulate their own problem solving by setting goals to meet needs, constructing plans to meet goals, and adjusting actions to complete plans. Each instructional phase poses a problem (What is my goal? What is my plan? What have I learned?) the student must solve by solving a series of smaller problems posed by the questions in each phase. The four questions differ from phase to phase but represent identical steps in the problem-solving sequence. That is, students answering the questions must: (1) identify the problem, (2) identify potential solutions to the problem, (3) identify barriers to solving the problem, and (4) identify consequences of each solution. These steps are fundamental in any problem-solving process, and they form the means–ends problem-solving sequence represented by the student questions in each phase and enable the student to solve the problem posed in that phase.

Figures 9.4, 9.5, and 9.6 provide worksheets to guide students as they address the questions in each phase, although these are intended simply as an example of the type of curricular support that could be developed to assist students to work through the questions in the model. As specified in Figure 9.4, an important outcome for the student will be to write a specific goal, which is identified in response to the fourth question (What can I do to make this happen?).

Figures 9.7, 9.8, and 9.9 are worksheets for use by the teacher in tracking which objectives associated with each student question have been addressed. Not every student will need instruction to match every objective, but teachers should be certain that students have the capacity to perform tasks associated with each objective, even if targeted instruction is not warranted.

An important feature of the SDLMI is that it acts as a feedback or monitoring loop that enables students to revise their action plan or goal based on their progress (Bandura, 1997). As students self-evaluate their progress toward their goal in phase 3, their determinations will dictate which option they pursue. If, for example, a student determines through her evaluation of the self-monitoring data that she is making sufficient progress toward the goal, she will continue to implement her action plan. If, however, she determines that her progress is not adequate, she has two courses of action. The first is to return to phase 2 and set a different action plan. This may mean changing the actual intervention to achieve the goal, or it may mean simply modifying the duration or intensity of the existing intervention strategy. If the student has already altered her action plan one or more times or believes that the action plan is adequate, the other option is to return to phase 1 and modify the goal. In most cases, this modification will narrow the goal or further define the

The Self-Determined Learning Model of Instruction (SDLMI):
Student Questions—*Phase 1, Set a Goal*

Name: _____ Date: _____

School: _____ (Date Phase 1 Began)

What is my goal? ☛*What class do you want to improve?*

☐ English
☐ Math
☐ Social studies
☐ Science
☐ Other:

☛ *Please answer below questions*

1. What do I want to learn or improve on in (   ) class?

_____

_____

_____

↓

2. What do I know about it now in (   ) class?

_____

_____

_____

↓

**3. What must change for me to learn what I don't know in (   )
class?**

_____

_____

_____

↓

4. What can I do to make this happen?

_____

_____

☛ *I have listed a specific, measurable activity for student question 4. This is my goal
in _____ class, the activity I will be working on during phase 2 and phase 3.*

End of phase 1 ↳ Go to phase 2

FIGURE 9.4. Student worksheet for SDLMI phase 1.

The Self-Determined Learning Model of Instruction (SDLMI):
Student Questions—*Phase 2, Take Action*

Name: _____ Date: _____

School: _____ (Date Phase 2 Began)

| **What is my plan?** ☛ Let's think about how to achieve the goal that you set. |

☛ *Please answer below questions*

5. What can I do to learn what I don't know?

_____

_____

_____

↓

6. What could keep me from taking action?

_____

_____

_____

↓

7. What can I do to remove these barriers?

_____

_____

_____

↓

8. When will I take action?

_____

_____

_____

☛ *End of phase 2. I will start working on my plan and then go on to phase 3.*

End of phase 2 ↳ Go to phase 3

FIGURE 9.5. Student worksheet for SDLMI phase 2.

The Self-Determined Learning Model of Instruction (SDLMI): Student Questions — *Phase 3, Adjust Goal or Plan*

Name: _____ Date: _____

School: _____ (Date Phase 3 Began)

> **What have I learned?** ☛ *Let's think about whether you achieved your goal or not.*

☛ *Please answer below questions*

9. What actions have I taken?

_____

_____

_____

↓

10. What barriers have been removed?

_____

_____

_____

↓

11. What has changed about what I don't know?

_____

_____

_____

↓

12. Do I know what I want to know?

_____

_____

_____

☛ **Did I achieve my goal?** *Please mark the square.* ☐ Yes ☐ No

If yes, *how do I feel about the results?* _____

_____

Now I will go to **phase 1** *and set a new goal.*

If no, *I will look at phase 1 again. If the goal is still a good one for me, I will move on to* **phase 2** *to revise my plan.* **Or** *I can rewrite my same goal or change it to a new goal.*

FIGURE 9.6. Student worksheet for SDLMI phase 3.

The Self-Determined Learning Model of Instruction:
Teacher Objectives and Educational Supports — *Phase 1, Set a Goal*

Teacher Name: _____   Date: _____

Student Name: _____   (Date Phase 1 Began)

☛ *Please mark (✓) on any educational supports you used.*

What is my goal? – Educational Supports

☐ Student self-assessment of interests, abilities, and instructional needs.
☐ Awareness training.
☐ Choice-making instruction.
☐ Problem-solving instruction.
☐ Decision-making instruction.
☐ Goal-setting instruction.

☛ *Please mark (✓) on teacher objectives that you met or targeted.*

Student Question 1: What do I want to learn? – Teacher Objectives

☐ Enable students to identify specific strengths and instructional needs.
☐ Enable students to communicate preferences, interests, beliefs, and values.
☐ Teach students to prioritize needs.

↓

Student Question 2: What do I know about it now? – Teacher Objectives

☐ Enable students to identify their current status in relation to the instructional need.
☐ Assist students to gather information about opportunities and barriers in their environments.

↓

Student Question 3: What must change for me to learn what I don't know? – Teacher Objectives

☐ Enable students to decide if action will be focused toward capacity building, modifying the environment, or both.
☐ Support students to choose a need to address from the prioritized list.

↓

Student Question 4: What can I do to make this happen? – Teacher Objectives

☐ Teach students to state a goal and identify criteria for achieving goal.

↳ Go to phase 2

FIGURE 9.7. Teacher guide for SDLMI phase 1.

The Self-Determined Learning Model of Instruction:
Teacher Objectives and Educational Supports — *Phase 2, Take Action*

Teacher Name: _____ Date: _____

Student Name: _____ (Date Phase 2 Began)

☛ *Please mark (✔) on any educational supports that you used.*

What is my plan? — Educational Supports	
☐ Self-scheduling.	☐ Problem-solving instruction.
☐ Self-instruction.	☐ Decision-making instruction.
☐ Antecedent cue regulation.	☐ Self-advocacy and assertiveness training.
☐ Choice-making instruction.	☐ Communication skills training.
☐ Goal-attainment strategies.	☐ Self-monitoring.

☛ *Please mark (✔) on teacher objectives that you met or targeted.*

Student Question 5: What can I do to learn what I don't know? — Teacher Objectives

☐ Enable students to self-evaluate current status and self-identified goal status.

↓

Student Question 6: What could keep me from taking action? — Teacher Objectives

☐ Enable students to determine plan of action to bridge gap between self-evaluated current status and self-identified goal status.

↓

Student Question 7: What can I do to remove these barriers? — Teacher Objectives

☐ Collaborate with student to identify most appropriate instructional strategies.
☐ Teach student needed student-directed learning strategies.
☐ Support student to implement student-directed learning strategies.
☐ Provide mutually agreed upon teacher-directed instruction.

↓

Student Question 8: When will I take action? — Teacher Objectives

☐ Enable student to determine schedule for action plan.
☐ Enable student to implement action plan.
☐ Enable student to self-monitor progress.

↳ Go to phase 3

FIGURE 9.8. Teacher guide for SDLMI phase 2.

The Self-Determined Learning Model of Instruction:
Teacher Objectives and Educational Supports—*Phase 3, Adjust Goal or Plan*

Teacher Name: _____ Date: _____

Student Name: _____ (Date Phase 3 Began)

☛ *Please mark (✓) on any educational supports that you used.*

What have I learned? — Educational Supports

☐ Self-evaluation strategies.
☐ Choice-making instruction.
☐ Goal-setting instruction.
☐ Problem-solving instruction.
☐ Decision-making instruction.
☐ Self-reinforcement strategies.
☐ Self-recording strategies.
☐ Self-monitoring.

☛ *Please mark (✓) on teacher objectives that you met or targeted.*

Student Question 9: What actions have I taken? — Teacher Objectives

☐ Enable student to self-evaluate progress toward goal achievement.

↓

Student Question 10: What barriers have been removed? — Teacher Objectives

☐ Collaborate with student to compare progress with desired outcomes.

↓

Student Question 11: What has changed about what I don't know? — Teacher Objectives

☐ Support student to reevaluate goal if progress is insufficient.
☐ Assist student to decide if goal remains the same or changes.
☐ Collaborate with student to identify if action plan is adequate or inadequate given revised or retained goal.
☐ Assist student to change action plan if necessary.

↓

Student Question 12: Do I know what I want to know? — Teacher Objectives

☐ Enable student to decide if progress is adequate, inadequate, or if goal has been achieved.

FIGURE 9.9. Teacher guide for SDLMI phase 3.

goal's focus, making it more achievable. The process becomes iterative, and every student should be theoretically able to modify his or her action plan or goal to the extent that he or she is able to attain the goal successfully. To this extent, the SDLMI can be grouped with similar self-regulated learning strategies that teach students to learn to adjust their goals and actions as a means to goal attainment (Graham & Harris, 1997).

Because the model itself is designed for teachers to implement, the language of the student questions is not intended to be understood by every student, nor does the model assume that students have life experiences that enable them fully to answer each question. The student questions are written in first-person voice in a relatively simple format with the intention that they are the starting point for discussion between the teacher and the student. Some students will learn and use all 12 questions as they are written. Other students will need to have the questions rephrased to be more understandable. Still other students, due to the intensity of their instructional needs, may need to have the teacher paraphrase the questions for them.

The first time a teacher uses the model with a student, the initial step in the implementation process is to read the question with or to the student, discuss what the question means, and, if necessary, change the wording to enable that student better to understand the intent of the question. Such wording changes must not change the problem-solving intent of the question. For example, changing student question 1 from "What do I want to learn?" to "What is my goal?" changes the nature of the question. The teacher objectives associated with each student question provide direction for possible wording changes. It is perhaps less important that actual changes in the words occur than that students take ownership of the process and adopt the question as their own instead of having questions imposed on them. Going through this process once, as the student progresses through the model, should result in a set of questions that a student accepts as his or her own.

TEACHER OBJECTIVES

The teacher objectives within the model are just that—the objectives a teacher will be trying to accomplish by implementing the model. In each instructional phase, the objectives are linked directly to the student questions. These objectives can be met by utilizing strategies provided in the educational supports section of the model. The teacher objectives provide a road map to assist the teacher to enable the student to solve the problem stated in the student question. For example, regarding the first student question (What do I want to learn?), teacher objectives linked to this question describe the activities in which students should be engaged in order to answer this question. In this case, it involves enabling students to identify their specific strengths and instructional needs; to identify and communicate their preferences, interests, beliefs, and values; and to prioritize their instructional needs. As teachers use the model, it is likely that they can generate more objectives that are relevant to the question, and they are encouraged to do so.

EDUCATIONAL SUPPORTS

The educational supports are not actually a part of the model but are what Joyce and Weil (1980) refer to as the model's syntax—how the model is implemented. Because the implementation of this model requires teachers to teach students to self-direct learning, we believe it is important to identify some strategies and supports that could be used to implement the model successfully. The majority of these supports are derived from the self-management literature and have been covered in previous chapters.

The emphasis in the model on the use of instructional strategies and educational supports that are student-directed provides another means of teaching students to teach themselves. As we have already indicated, teaching students to use the student questions will teach them a self-regulated problem-solving strategy. Concurrently, teaching students to use various student-directed learning strategies provides students with another layer of skills that enables them to become causal agents in their own lives.

As important as it is to utilize the student-directed learning strategies, not every instructional strategy implemented will be student-directed. The purpose of any model of teaching is to promote student learning and growth. There are circumstances in which the most effective instructional method or strategy to achieve a particular educational outcome will be a teacher-directed strategy. Students who are considering what plan of action to implement to achieve a self-selected goal can recognize that teachers have expertise in instructional strategies and take full advantage of that expertise.

VALIDATION OF THE SDLMI

We have conducted research with students with intellectual and developmental disabilities to determine the efficacy of the model. The fundamental purpose of any model of instruction is to promote student learning. Teachers use models of instruction to drive curriculum and assessment development and to design instructional methods, materials, and strategies, all with the intent of improving the quality of the instructional experience and, presumably, enhancing student achievement. Thus, the first requirement of any model of instruction is that teachers can use the model to teach students educationally valid skills or concepts.

Wehmeyer, Palmer, Agran, Mithaug, and Martin (2000) conducted a field test of the SDLMI with 21 teachers in two states responsible for the instruction of adolescents receiving special education services who identified a total of 40 students with intellectual disabilities, learning disabilities, or emotional or behavioral disorders. The efficacy of the model to enable students to achieve educationally valid goals was examined using the Goal Attainment Scaling (GAS) process, which measures student goal attainment compared with a teacher expectation of progress determined at the time the goal was set. In addition to this indicator, we also collected pre- and postintervention data regarding student self-determination using The Arc's Self-Determination Scale (Wehmeyer, 1996), a student self-report measure of self-determination, and administered a questionnaire examining student goal orientation.

The field test indicated that the model was effective in enabling students to attain educationally valid goals. From a total of 43 distinct goals, teachers rated 55% of the goals on which students received instruction as having been achieved as expected or exceeding expectations. Of the remainder, teachers indicated that students made progress on an additional 25% of their goals, without fully achieving them, and only 20% of the goals were rated as indicating no student progress. Additionally, there were significant differences in pre- and postintervention scores on self-determination, with postintervention scores more positive than preintervention scores.

Agran, Blanchard, and Wehmeyer (2000) used a delayed multiple-baseline-across-three-groups design to examine the efficacy of the SDLMI for adolescents with severe disabilities. Students collaborated with their teachers to implement the first phase of the model and, as a result, identified one goal as a target behavior. Prior to implementing phase 2 of the model, teachers and researchers collected baseline data on student performance of these goals. At staggered intervals subsequent to baseline data collection, teachers implemented the model with students, and data collection continued through the end of instructional activities and into a maintenance phase. As was the case with the field test, Agran and colleagues (2000) also collected data about goal attainment using the GAS procedure.

As before, the model enabled teachers to teach students educationally valid goals. The mean GAS score for the total sample was 60, indicating that, on average, students exceeded teachers' expectations for achievement of their goals. (A score of 50 on the GAS indicates that students achieved goals at the level expected, satisfactorily. Scores below 40 indicate less than expected progress, and those of 60 and above represent higher levels of goal attainment than expected.) In total, 17 of the 19 participants achieved their personal goals at or above the teacher-rated expected outcome levels. Only two students were rated as indicating no progress on their goals.

Similarly, McGlashing-Johnson, Agran, Sitlington, Cavin, and Wehmeyer (2003) examined the effects of the SDLMI on the job performance of four students with moderate to severe cognitive disabilities who ranged from 16 to 21 years of age and participated in a work-based learning program in the community as part of their transition programs, using a multiple-baseline-across-participants design. Three of the four participants achieved their self-selected goals, and one student did not meet the mastery criterion but performed at a higher level during the training condition than in baseline. Agran et al. (2006) investigated the effects of the SDLMI on the academic skill performance of three junior high school students with intellectual disabilities, finding that all students could achieve goals linked to the general education curriculum.

Finally, Palmer and Wehmeyer (2003) examined the efficacy of the model with elementary-age (K–3) students with disabilities. Fourteen teachers from two states were recruited to implement the SDLMI with 50 students who were identified as having a disability or at risk for such. The mean GAS score was 52.90 (ranging from 30 to 70), indicating that students achieved goals at an acceptable level. Students also showed gains in knowledge about goal setting, and teachers indicated they found the process effective for teaching students.

PART IV

CURRICULUM MODIFICATIONS
AND STUDENT INVOLVEMENT

CHAPTER 10

Technology and Universal Design to Promote Self-Determination

To this point, we have focused on teacher- and student-mediated/self-directed strategies to promote the self-determination of students with intellectual and developmental disabilities. An area of considerable potential and a growing evidence base with regard to the education of learners with intellectual disabilities involves technology-mediated instruction. Specifically, the Individuals with Disabilities Education Act (IDEA) requires that the Individualized Eduation Programs (IEP) of all students with disabilities consider whether the students need assistive technology. IDEA also requires that the IEP of students with disabilities promote involvement with and access to the general education curriculum. As discussed in Chapter 1, promoting self-determination should be part of efforts to achieve access to the general education curriculum. There is a growing consensus that to achieve that access for all students, educators will have to apply principals of universal design for learning.

In this chapter, we examine the role technology can play in instruction, look at the principles of universal design (UD) and its application to learning, discuss issues of cognitive accessibility that need to be addressed to enable learners with intellectual and developmental disabilities to utilize technology, and overview the literature pertaining to the impact of technology use on education outcomes and self-determination for this population.

UNIVERSAL DESIGN

Before discussing technology use by students with intellectual and developmental disabilities and its application to promote self-determination, we turn first to issues pertaining to universal design. Technology has the potential to enhance self-determination, promote greater independence, and enhance learning for students with disabilities, but only if they can use it. Principles of UD address accessibility issues.

The principles of UD emerged from the field of architecture, where, as applied to buildings and built environments, they suggest that all buildings/environments should be accessible to all people. These principles were subsequently applied to the design and development of consumer products and assistive devices with the same intent. In essence, the principle of UD was introduced to ensure that members of certain groups have access to the environment or products that can enhance their quality of life. Buildings are designed with adequate ramps, wider doors, and accessible restrooms, and products are designed with simple controls and clearly perceptible uses. These principles, as applied to technology design and development, provide many of the keys to addressing the underutilization of technology by people with intellectual and developmental disabilities by focusing on the features of technology that address user characteristics. The Center for Universal Design (1997) has identified seven principles of universal design to consider when designing technology. These are:

1. *Equitable use*: A design is useful and marketable to any group of users.
2. *Flexibility in use*: A design accommodates a wide range of individual preferences and abilities.
3. *Simple and intuitive use*: Use of the design is easy to understand, regardless of user's experience, knowledge, or language or cognitive skills.
4. *Perceptible information*: The design communicates the information needed by the user, through different modes or by providing adequate contrast.
5. *Tolerance for error*: The design minimizes adverse consequences or accidental or unintended actions.
6. *Low physical effort*: The design can be used comfortably with minimum fatigue.
7. *Size and space for approach and use appropriate*: Design allows for approach, reach, manipulation, and device use independent of user's body size, posture, or mobility.

Barriers to Technology Use for Students with Intellectual and Developmental Disabilities

Characteristics of learners with intellectual disabilities include impairments in memory, language use and communication, abstract conceptualization, generalization, and problem identification/problem solving, as well as physical and sensory impairments, all of which affect students' capacity to utilize technology-based educational supports. Following, these characteristics are discussed within the context of their impact on technology use so as to provide educators with a sense of how to evaluate technology for its utility for students with intellectual and developmental disabilities.

Memory and Ease of Operation

Technology interfaces are often complex, as developers seek to provide users with a wide array of program features, but their complexity often renders them unusable by students with intellectual disabilities. For example, students with memory impairments may not be able to recall multistep operations or navigate menu structures. Interfaces should be intuitive, without overwhelming students with too many options. Often, it is better to provide a single, consistent approach to performing a program function. For example, in most Windows-based word processing programs, computer users can copy and paste text in a variety of ways: highlighting the text and selecting "Copy" and then "Paste" from the text toolbar or dropdown menu; highlighting the text and clicking on the "Copy" icon on the toolbar, followed by the "Paste" icon; or highlighting text and right clicking on it, then selecting "Copy" and "Paste" from that menu. Such a range of options may be too complex for some students with intellectual disabilities, for whom it may be simpler to stick to one modality (e.g., using the icons on the toolbar) across multiple task activities. In general, devices that require users to memorize long sequences of commands to succeed present barriers for students with intellectual disabilities.

Language and Communication

The language involved in technology use is often not consistent with that of everyday communication. Terminology used in some technology systems can be complex and may introduce new definitions for common terms. For example, a menu in a computer program, while conceptually similar (an array of choices) to a menu at a restaurant, may confuse a student with intellectual disability. Use of terms with multiple meanings and abstract metaphors (e.g., files, folders) can pose barriers to students with intellectual disabilities, who respond to language based on a more literal, concrete view of the world.

The assumption by technology developers that all users can read introduces an even more significant obstacle to technology use by students with intellectual and developmental disabilities. Although the technology field is increasingly embracing the use of more universally accepted graphics to communicate information, most software and devices continue to rely primarily on text to present program options and provide instructions to users.

Conceptualization Skills and Abstract Thinking

It is likely that most students with intellectual disabilities will have some level of difficulty understanding the abstract concepts and metaphors used in technology. An example above referred to the use of the file-and-folder metaphor. Beyond the need to conceive of virtual files and folders, computer users must also conceptualize the virtual location of these files within a computer directory.

Other technologies present their own challenges to the capacity of students with cognitive impairments to think abstractly. Communication devices often include customizable picture or text buttons that, when pressed, speak the indicated word or phrase. To provide added functionality, most of these devices include a feature that allows the user to create different overlays, or layers, so that more words or phrases can be accessed. For example, a typical device may have 16 buttons that each can be programmed to speak a designated phrase, but an additional switch might allow the user to activate another layer of programming so that the same 16 buttons speak entirely different phrases. Many of these devices are not usable by students with intellectual disabilities due, in part, to inability to conceive of these different layers.

Other examples may be as simple as failure to recognize or understand the meaning of when the mouse arrow turns into a hand icon when placed over a clickable element of a website or not understanding the difference between a single click, a double click, and a right click. Even the most basic software features—such as buttons being disabled or grayed out when they have no practical use—often are too subtle to be recognized by users with cognitive disabilities. In summary, there seems to be an inherent tendency in technology development to add more features to a system or device. The result is usually an interface that requires relatively a high level of cognitive ability to navigate the system.

Problem Identification and Problem Solving

Using technology on a regular basis often requires problem identification and problem solving by the technology user, areas in which students with intellectual and developmental disabilities may have difficulty. This difficulty may be due to typical learning curves related to the acquisition of knowledge and skills to use a program or device, lack of experience with the technology, excessive complexity, poor interface design, program or system bugs and failures, conflicts with other technology, or other situations. Technology users rely on their ability to generalize previous learning to problem solve unexpected occurrences, but many students with intellectual disabilities have limited ability to generalize learning from one situation to another and, therefore, do not develop the strategies that typical users of technology develop to overcome problems.

The principles of universal design illustrate some of the features that teachers can evaluate to determine the utility of technology for a student. If all technology devices took into account all of the principles of universal design, it is quite likely that many more of them would be usable by students with intellectual and developmental disabilities. Several such principles are particularly important to students with intellectual and developmental disabilities and warrant specific mention. First, devices that abide by the principle of flexibility in use inherently accommodate for use by a wider range of individual preferences and abilities, for example by providing options that accommodate for accuracy and precision or adapt to a user's pace. Computer programs providing multiple input and output options (auditory, visual, icon, etc.) fit this category, as do telephones that have larger buttons, with more space in between numbers (Center for Universal Design, 1997).

Issues of simplicity and intuitiveness of use are also obviously important for people with intellectual disabilities. Many devices are overly complex and operate counter to users' expectations, including common items such as VCRs and alarm clocks. Universally designed devices also typically provide some supports (prompting, graphic, visual, or audio directions) for use. The principle of perceptible information requires not only that information needed to operate the device be easily seen, but also that such information be provided in multiple modes and redundantly.

Finally, an important and often overlooked UD feature for people with intellectual and developmental disabilities is the principle of tolerance for error. People with cognitive, sensory, and physical impairments frequently make mistakes in using technology; if those errors result in failed use, the device becomes essentially impossible for people with intellectual disability to access. For example, irons that shut off automatically minimize the risk of error associated with using an iron (Center for Universal Design, 1997). Developing technology that never results in unexpected errors is essentially impossible. Given the difficulty many persons with disabilities have responding to unexpected errors, it is imperative that priority be placed on identifying highly reliable technology supports for students with intellectual disability. Device failure is often a function of device complexity. The more complex a device is and the more features it has, the more likely it is to have unexpected errors. At times, it may be more important to identify less complex devices with fewer features if they provide the benefit of greater reliability. Moreover, many devices have, in essence, a one-strike-and-you're-out policy, where one error (e.g., wrong key stroke) results in the failure of the user's session. For example, the value of a dialogue box that prompts you to confirm a selection (e.g., deletion, exit) becomes evident when you inadvertently hit the "Exit" icon without having saved your work. The dialogue box allows you to select "Cancel" and does not immediately delete unsaved work. Students with intellectual and developmental disabilities need devices that minimize the potential for error and allow errors to occur without dire consequences.

Universal Design for Learning

A recent outgrowth of the emphasis on UD is the application of this notion to educational settings and, particularly, to the development and delivery of instructional materials, referred to as universal design for learning (UDL). Orkwis and McLane (1998) defined UDL as "the design of instructional materials and activities that allows the learning goals to be achievable by individuals with wide differences in their abilities to see, hear, speak, move, read, write, understand English, attend, organize, engage, and remember" (p. 9). When those learning goals include instruction to promote self-determination, the use of accessible materials becomes critically important.

To this point, we have discussed the potential impact technology can have on the lives of students with intellectual and developmental disabilities. The remainder of the chapter (drawing on Wehmeyer, Smith, and Davies, 2005, and Wehmeyer, Smith, Palmer, Davies, and Stock, 2004) discusses how technology has been and can be used to promote self-determination and its component elements.

TECHNOLOGY USE TO PROMOTE SELF-DETERMINATION

Promoting Access

Teaching anything, including self-determination, begins with student access to educational content, materials, and pedagogy. Technology can promote greater access to educational content and inclusive practices for students with intellectual and developmental disabilities (Foshay & Ludlow, 2006). A comprehensive review of technology as applied to instruction is beyond the scope of this chapter or this text, but in many cases technology to promote access to education and learning can help foster self-determination even when the technology is not directly teaching component elements of self-determined behavior. Foshay and Ludlow (2006, p. 103) observed:

> Computer users make decisions when interacting with computer operating systems, with software applications, and with hardware input devices such as a mouse, keyboard, switch, or microphone. Computer software provides many opportunities for choice making. Successful manipulation of dialog boxes, menu commands, or navigation in and around a program or web site may lead to enhanced feelings of control and self-direction. For example, creating a holiday card using a computer program requires a student to choose pictures, font color, style, and size, as well as the card's message. This experience of creating a custom made card may result in feelings of self-efficacy, self-worth, and independence.

As such, an examination of technology use to promote self-determination involves looking at technology that promotes access to education and learning. Using technology effectively in educational settings requires successful operation of all related hardware, the applicable operating system, one or more software programs, and so forth. Barriers can exist at any or all of these points in the system, and any one of them might make the entire system inaccessible to students with cognitive disabilities. Access begins at the operating system level. Fortunately, companies building operating systems have made progress in providing accessibility options within their systems. These generally involve user-controlled features related to use of the keyboard, mouse, and display, which can be adjusted to facilitate access. While most of these features target students with vision, hearing, or physical impairments, several are also useful to students with intellectual disabilities. For example, Microsoft's Windows XP includes a series of features primarily for people with physical disabilities called StickyKeys, ToggleKeys, and FilterKeys. FilterKeys can be used to cancel consecutive keystrokes and play a sound when a key has been successfully struck. Other examples include SoundSentry (which provides on-screen cues when computer sounds are made), controls to adjust the display contrast and font size, and keyboard controls for mouse movement.

Palmtop and Other Platforms

Palmtop computers are becoming more and more prevalent in daily life. These devices have a variety of features that make them more user-friendly than traditional desktop systems, including touch-screen interfaces (that replace mouse and keyboard use) and built-in audio-recording and playback capacity. Additionally, their portability provides the potential for powerful, computer-aided assistance in a wide variety of community settings, and their use of mainstream hardware platforms has the potential to keep costs down compared to the high cost of dedicated assistive technology hardware devices.

Some characteristics of palmtop computers, however, tend to be barriers to students with intellectual and developmental disabilities. For one, the variety of such devices is confusing, with software interfaces requiring fairly sophisticated conceptualization, learning, and retention skills. Another barrier is the relatively small touch screen. While touch-screen interfaces often have a high level of intuitiveness (i.e., directly tapping on a desired option without having to navigate there with a mouse), the limited availability of display space requires software developers to provide controls and other tappable areas that are extremely small. This allows many features and options to be displayed on the screen at any time but limits access for students with intellectual disabilities due to the cluttered screen and the need for very precise tapping.

Several approaches for simplifying access can be used. Pocket Voyager, developed by AbleLink Technologies (www.ablelinktech.com), is a program designed to improve access to palmtop computers specifically for people with intellectual and developmental disabilities. The application "sits on top" of the mainstream palmtop operating system to provide a simplified user interface (see Figure 10.1). When this software is launched on a palmtop computer, the buttons and controls on the hardware unit are either deactivated or reprogrammed such that when one is pressed, the system automatically returns to the familiar Pocket Voyager interface. In addition, an interface is provided for teachers to create large, multimedia buttons on screen for any application loaded on to the palmtop computer. The only icons/controls that appear on screen are the ones created in this way, eliminating

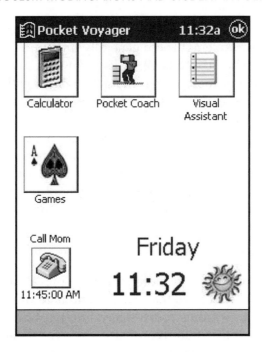

FIGURE 10.1. Pocket Voyager customizable desktop.

much of the potential for confusion and unintended activation of programs. To set up an on-screen multimedia button, teachers can designate a custom picture or icon to display on the button and record an audio message that further identifies its purpose ("Tap here again if you want to play solitaire"). When the multimedia button is first tapped, the device plays the identifying message; when it is tapped again, the designated application launches. To enable access further, buttons created on screen in Pocket Voyager are large enough to be tapped by the user's finger, forgoing the need for a stylus.

Stock, Davies, Davies, and Wehmeyer (2006) evaluated the Pocket Voyager interface to determine if it made navigation of palmtop computer features more accessible to users with intellectual disabilities. Participants completed a structured set of navigation/computer tasks using both the experimental and control conditions. Measurements included the amount of assistance needed and the number of errors made in completing the tasks. Participants with intellectual disabilities made significantly fewer errors and required significantly fewer prompts while using the specialized software interface in comparison to when using the standard Windows CE operating system interface.

Input Devices

Although new platforms are increasingly available, the desktop computer remains the most common system with which students interact, and the computer keyboard and mouse remain the most typical input devices. On the surface, basic mouse use seems fairly straightforward: you see something on the screen and click on it. Many students with intellectual or developmental disabilities, however, do not intuitively pick up on the spatial orientation requirements of mouse operation and may need some instruction. In fact, students with intellectual and developmental disabilities may need explicit instruction in most basic computer skills, including mouse and keyboard use and turning the computer on and off.

Davies, Stock, and Wehmeyer (2004) conducted a study to examine the use of a multimedia software program designed for self-directed computer training and skill assessment of people with intellectual disabilities. Nine adults with intellectual disabilities who had never used a computer before were taught mouse use, computer navigation, and keyboard skills using the software program. All participants significantly increased their computer skills from baseline in a self-directed manner.

Keyboard use is largely dependent on a person's literacy skills, often a barrier for students with intellectual disabilities. Additionally, keyboards require a degree of fine-motor control, visual-perception skills, and the ability to understand multistep concepts (e.g., CONTROL + ALT + DELETE). Alternative keyboards and keyboard overlays have been developed primarily to address physical access issues, and some have been designed to improve access for young children whose cognitive skills have not yet fully developed or for use with specialized hardware or software.

Keyboards are used for entry of content and for navigation (e.g., use of text menus to access controls and features). Emerging voice recognition systems, such as ScanSoft's Dragon Dictate and IBM's ViaVoice, hold promise for addressing barriers to keyboard use for some students with intellectual disabilities. These systems allow users both to control computer navigation (e.g., "open Microsoft Word") and to provide content input (e.g., write letters). As is typical of most powerful computing technologies, however, the complex user interfaces that have been developed to provide access to the wide array of available features in voice recognition systems pose a barrier to individuals with cognitive disabilities. An option for students with intellectual disabilities may be a scaled-down version that provides a simplified, consistent interface at the expense of eliminating some features.

Touch screens, which are becoming increasingly popular in some specialized computer systems, such as in shopping mall or university kiosks, provide an opportunity to improve access to computers for students with intellectual disabilities. Essentially, a touch screen can provide many of the same functions as a computer mouse, but without having to make the cognitive connection between mouse and cursor movement. Touch screens do have limitations in terms of advanced inputs like double clicking and the drag-and-drop interface.

Internet Access and Browser Use

Finally, with regard to promoting access, the potential of the Internet and the World Wide Web to benefit students with intellectual disabilities seems particularly promising, but like other aspects of computer and software access, Internet access is restricted for many people with intellectual disabilities. For a variety of reasons, many of them discussed earlier, browsers currently used to access the web are not usable by most students with intellectual disabilities.

Researchers and developers at AbleLink Technologies (Davies, Stock, & Wehmeyer, 2001) developed a web browser called Web Trek (depicted in Figure 10.2) that was cognitively accessible to users with intellectual disabilities. The browser was designed to provide an accessible interface to support these users to perform the most common Internet tasks, such as entering a URL, searching the Internet, and saving and returning to favorite sites. The browser contains several features to ensure accessibility:

- *Audio prompts.* Two types of audio prompt are used. The first is a type of "button talk," whereby a message is played describing the use of a button when the cursor arrow is placed over it (without clicking). This is similar to the balloon help that displays the name or function of a button when the mouse is moved over it in most Windows applications. The second is "error minimization" cueing, in which a message is played following a user-

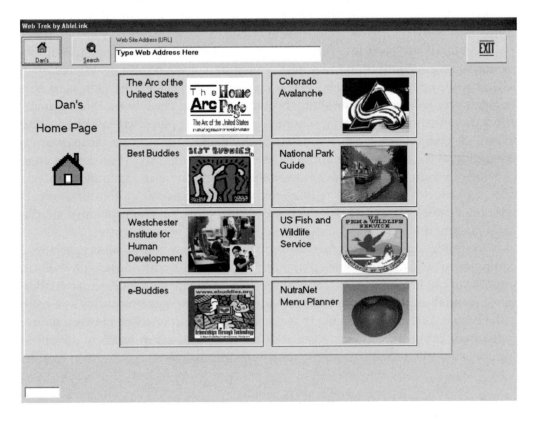

FIGURE 10.2. Web Trek browser.

initiated event (e.g., a click) to guide the user to the next-most-likely step in a task.

- *Reduced screen clutter.* Only basic features are provided in the Web Trek interface, minimizing screen clutter. Also, buttons and other on-screen features are only displayed when they have a use, as opposed to being grayed out.
- *Personalization and customization.* Web Trek displays the user's name on the home button and homepage as well as a digital picture of the user. In addition, buttons and controls can be displayed or hidden based on the needs of the particular user.
- *Use of graphics.* Web Trek uses a picture-based search process. To provide enhanced direction, graphics or buttons are provided in combination with audio prompts that reference the graphic.
- *Error minimization methodologies.* This broad category of features includes anything that reduces opportunities or chances for making errors. Examples include everything listed above, as well as design considerations such as consistent placement of familiar buttons from screen to screen and automating steps when possible.

Adolescents with intellectual disabilities were able to use Web Trek to select websites and to navigate to preferred sites with greater independence and fewer errors than when using a typical browser (Internet Explorer) (Davies et al., 2001). Further, all participants reported that it was a positive experience and demonstrated their enjoyment by asking to do so again. Participants were interested in the results of their Internet searches; in all instances they were able to find information about and pictures related to the topics they searched for. Every participant expressed a desire either to continue after the evaluation session was over or to return to continue another day (Davies et al., 2001).

Promoting Independence and Decreasing Dependence

Access to educational technology ensures that students benefit from the secondary impact of technology to promote self-determination. At the next level down, though still not at the level of using technology explicitly to teach skills pertaining to self-determination, is the use of technology to promote independence and decrease dependence. The former typically involves using technology to teach independent living, community integration, and similar skills. The latter involves the use of prompting technologies that provide external supports and replace the need for other people to provide those supports. We have intentionally not focused on assistive technologies like communication or mobility devices in this chapter unless they have been applied to promote specific self-determination skills. These powerful devices can increase independence, but a comprehensive examination of them is simply beyond the scope of this effort. Nevertheless, students who need communication, mobility, hearing, or vision assistive technology should receive it, and these technologies can contribute to the development of a student's self-determination.

Promoting Independence

Technology has been used to promote independence in a number of ways. Branham, Collins, Schuster, and Kleinert (1999) used a combination of classroom simulation and video-based modeling to augment community-based instruction that taught students with moderate intellectual disabilities a range of functional skills, including mailing a letter, cashing a check, and crossing the street. Lancioni, O'Reilly, Oliva, and Coppa (2001) used a microswitch that could be operated through vocalizations that enabled children with multiple disabilities to operate environmental control devices (e.g., turning on and off lights).

Davies, Stock, and Wehmeyer (2003a) taught nine adults with intellectual disabilities how to use a local ATM with a program simulating ATM use. Participants were pretested on their ability to use an ATM and, after a brief training period, tested again. Participants required significantly fewer help prompts and made fewer errors when operating the real ATM after training.

Nutrition, cooking, and food-related functional tasks have been the frequent target of technology-mediated instruction for students with intellectual and developmental disabilities. Trask-Tyler, Grossi, and Heward (1994) taught three students with developmental disabilities and visual impairments how to cook three different meals following tape-recorded instructions. Lancioni, Oliva, Pellegrino, and Soresi (1998) used a similar system to teach a man with intellectual disability cooking-related skills. Katz, Johnson, and Dalby (1981) taught food-group discrimination to adults with intellectual and developmental disabilities using slide presentations.

Langone and colleagues have engaged in a series of studies that utilized multimedia instructional technology to teach grocery-shopping skills to students with intellectual and developmental disabilities. Langone, Shade, Clees, and Day (1999) examined the effectiveness of a multimedia instructional program to affect the generalization of match-to-sample skills of students with intellectual disabilities to a grocery store setting. The multimedia program included photographs depicting target stimuli (e.g., cereal boxes as they appear on grocery store shelves) in an attempt to increase the likelihood that the selection of specified cereal boxes would generalize to grocery stores in the community. Their findings strongly suggested that discriminations established in a multimedia instructional setting generalized to the community-based grocery store. Similarly, Mechling, Gast, and Langone (2002) showed that students who learned functional words found in grocery stores using computer-based video instruction generalized the learned words to the actual setting.

Finally, Haring and colleagues have used videotape modeling to teach general purchasing skills to students with autism and intellectual disabilities. Haring, Kennedy, Adams, and Pitts-Conway (1987) showed that students who learned to purchase items from three different stores using videotaped training could successfully do so. Similarly, Haring, Breen, Weiner, Kennedy, and Bednersh (1995) taught six students with intellectual disabilities purchasing skills through the same process.

Employment and vocational education are areas in which technology has been applied to improve the independence of people with intellectual and developmental disabilities. Wehmeyer and colleagues (2006) conducted a meta-analysis of single-subject–design studies examining the use of technology in employment-related activities for people with intellectual disabilities and found that the use of technology to promote outcomes in this area was shown to be generally effective, in particular when universal design features were addressed. For example, Davies, Stock, and Wehmeyer (2003b) evaluated a system that was designed to provide vocational supports for individuals with intellectual disabilities. This system, which involved self-directed audio and video prompts on a Windows CE–based handheld computer, was evaluated in an employment setting to determine its utility for improving task accuracy and independence on two vocational assembly tasks: folding pizza boxes and packaging a commercial software product. Ten individuals with intellectual disabilities performed each task with and without the presence of the technology system. After initial training on both the task and use of the computer system, participants used the specialized software to follow step-by-step picture and audio prompts at their own pace. Results indicated that the computerized prompting system significantly improved task performance. In addition, these gains were achieved with significantly greater independence, as measured by the amount of assistance required from a job coach to complete each task, and participants expressed positive reactions to as well as preference for using the specialized prompting system.

Decreasing Dependence

An area of growth in knowledge about how technology can promote self-determination is in the area of technologies designed to provide prompting support to people who require it and to reduce or eliminate the need for others to provide prompts, thus reducing the dependency of people with intellectual and developmental disabilities on others. For example, Davies, Stock, and Wehmeyer (2002a) evaluated the impact of a palmtop PC-based software program, Visual Assistant, used by students to support learning through antecedent cue regulation, self-instruction, and self-monitoring/evaluation strategies. Visual Assistant is a multi-media software program designed to run on a Windows CE platform that allows users to view step-by-step picture sequences along with audio instructions at their own pace. Audio instructions and digital pictures can be created to customize the system. Activities are task-analyzed according to the training and support needs of each user. Digital pictures and audio instructions are then downloaded for each step in the task. Each task can be represented on the palmtop screen with an icon that users press to initiate instructions. After a task is selected, the picture for the first step is displayed and the first audio instruction is played. After completing the step, the user presses the "Done" button, which loads the next picture, and the "Play" button to hear the associated audio instruction.

Davies and colleagues (2002a) examined the use of Visual Assistant with 10 participants with intellectual disabilities receiving community-based vocational supports or enrolled in a community-based transition program. Participants were less dependent (requiring fewer external prompts) and more productive (making fewer errors) when using the program. Riffel and colleagues (2005) showed that teaching adolescents with intellectual disabilities to use Visual Assistant in completing transition-related tasks resulted in students requiring fewer prompts to complete the tasks and increased the number of steps that they completed independently.

Lancioni and colleagues have examined the ability of audio- and video-based prompting systems to reduce dependence and increase independence. For example, Lancioni, van den Hof, Boelens, Rocha, and Seedhouse (1998) evaluated the efficacy of a computer-based system designed to provide audio, visual (pictorial), and vibratory prompts to assist users with task steps. Three adults with intellectual and developmental disabilities used the system to improve their percentage of correct performances on tasks, even when compared with a strictly card-based prompting system. Mechling and Gast (1997) used an audio- and video-based prompting system, an augmentative communication device with picture overlays and recorded speech, to support students with intellectual disabilities to perform multistep tasks at a higher rate of independence.

TECHNOLOGY USE TO PROMOTE COMPONENT ELEMENTS OF SELF-DETERMINED BEHAVIOR

Technology can be used both to teach students skills promoting self-determination and to enable students with intellectual and developmental disabilities to use those skills.

Making Choices and Expressing Preferences

As covered, making choices and expressing preferences are important component elements of self-determined behavior. Obviously, any alternative or augmentative communication device should enable the user to communicate his or her preferences. Several studies have also specifically examined the efficacy of using microswitches to express preferences and make choices. Wacker, Wiggins, Fowler, and Berg (1988) conducted a series of studies showing that students with severe multiple disabilities could learn to use microswitches to express preferences. In one study, students learned to express their preference for a toy by pressing a microswitch. In another, students learned to press a switch to activate a tape recorder that played a message indicating the student had a specific request. Singh and colleagues (2003) taught a child with severe multiple disabilities to use microswitch technology to communicate her preference of what to eat or drink.

Solving Problems and Making Decisions

Research has shown technology to be effective in teaching students problem-solving and decision-making skills. Margalit (1991, 1995) evaluated the efficacy of a social skills–training computer program titled I Found a Solution that presented 24 computer-generated interpersonal conflict scenarios. Students who were trained to analyze social situations involving interpersonal conflict were subsequently rated as having greater cooperation skills and more effective self-control. Woodward, Carnine, and Gersten (1988) examined the effectiveness of computer simulations of health-related problems to teach problem solving. Students with cognitive disabilities were randomly assigned to one of two groups; both received direct, structured instruction, but one also participated in computer simulation activities. Students in the computer simulation group had significantly better problem-solving skills than the structured teaching-only group.

Davies, Stock, and Wehmeyer (2003b) used a modified version of Visual Assistant to provide decision-making support. This software, Pocket Compass, is a portable multimedia application that operates on the Pocket PC palmtop computer platform and utilizes customized picture and audio prompts to guide users through the decision-making process. The process works as a typical prompt device, showing pictures (and providing audio prompts) sequentially as students progress through the task. At decision points, up to four pictures can be set to display on the screen at once, each representing a different choice. With the images displayed, audio instructions that relate to the set of images play (e.g., "Touch the picture on screen that matches the number shown on the second page of the invoice"). Depending upon which picture is tapped, the system then follows the corresponding sequence of picture and audio cues through to the next decision point or to completion. The audio instructions and associated picture cues help the user make proper choices given relevant environmental data. Participants in the research, 40 adolescents and adults with intellectual disabilities, made fewer decision-point errors when using the system, required fewer prompts to complete tasks, and were able to perform more complex tasks than previously.

Promoting Self-Direction and Student-Directed Learning

Most of the prompting technologies described in this chapter constitute the application of technology to promote self-direction. Palmtop PC–based technology, such as the Visual Assistant and Pocket Compass programs, enable students to self-regulate task performance and learning through antecedent cue regulation, self-instruction (albeit with instructions coming from the device and not the individual), and self-monitoring (selecting "Done"). Davies and colleagues (2002b) found that adolescents and adults with intellectual disabilities were able to engage in time management activities in a self-directed manner using an automated, audio-based schedule-prompting software system operating from a Palmtop PC platform.

SUMMARY

Technology has the potential to enable people to become much more self-determined. To date, too few applications have been developed for and evaluated with people with intellectual and developmental disabilities, in part because many devices are not cognitively accessible. There is, however, a sufficient database suggesting that technology devices can enable students with intellectual and developmental disabilities to become more independent and to perform activities like expressing preferences, making choices, solving problems, and self-regulating task performance, all of which enable students to be more self-determined.

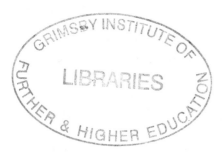

CHAPTER 11

Student Involvement
in Educational Planning

The Individuals with Disabilities Education Act (IDEA) mandates special education and related services to prepare children with disabilities for further education, employment, and independent living. This mandate is achieved through the development of an Individualized Education Program (IEP). The IEP of each child with a disability who is at least 16 years old (14 years old in many states; Grack, 2005) must identify transition services that will facilitate the student's transition from school to postsecondary education, employment, and/or independent living. These transition goals and activities must be based on students' needs while considering their interests, skills, and limits as identified by student-expressed interests, transition assessment, and parental input (Johnson, 2005). The IEP meeting and (often more specifically) the transition-planning meeting is an important vehicle to enable students both to learn and to practice skills that enable them to become more self-determined. Student involvement in educational planning is a critical component of efforts to promote self-determination. This chapter examines the knowledge base pertaining to student involvement, explores the importance of considering student diversity in the planning process, and covers existing approaches to promote student involvement.

RESEARCH ON STUDENT INVOLVEMENT IN IEP MEETINGS

O'Brien, O'Brien, and Mount (1997) suggested that professionals dominated the IEP planning discussions. To address partially the lack of student input, federal special education law now requires that students be invited to attend their IEP meetings if transition services are to be discussed so that the educational planning reflects and is driven by student postschool interests and preferences. The invitation implies that students are intended to be actively involved in IEP meeting discussions, and IEP involvement begins with students attending their IEP meetings.

Over the last few years, research shows, an increasing number of students have attended their IEP meetings. Vac and colleagues (1985) reported in a direct observation study that 4% of students attended their IEP meetings. Williams and O'Leary (2001) proposed that that many schools did not invite students to attend their IEP meetings, and as a result students seldom attended. Martin, Greene, and Borland (2004) conducted a statewide survey of building and special education administrators, who indicated that students almost always receive invitations to their IEP meetings; most reported that students attended their meetings some-to-most of the time. Martin, Marshall, and Sale (2004) found through analyzing post-IEP meeting survey results that students attend almost 70% of their meetings. Cameto, Levine, and Wagner (2004) found in their national survey that parents and school staff reported 94% of their children or students attended their IEP meetings. Martin, Van Dycke, Greene, and colleagues (2006), while observing 109 secondary IEP meetings, found that 78% of the students attended at least a portion of their IEP meetings. But does attendance enable students to serve as equal IEP team members?

Students who attended typical educator-directed IEP meetings often reported that they did not know what to do, did not understand the purpose of the meeting or what was said, and felt as if none of the adult participants listened to them when they spoke (Lehmann, Bassett, & Sands, 1999; Lovitt, Cushing, & Stump, 1994; Morningstar, Turnbull, & Turnbull, 1995; Powers, Turner, Matuszewski, Wilson, & Loesch, 1999). When students attended these traditional educator-directed IEP meetings, they simply served as token members and faced educational harm, as the intimidating process seemed to instill in them a sense of educational disillusionment (Lehman et al., 1999; Powers et al., 1999).

More recently, over 3 consecutive years, Martin, Marshall, and Sale (2004) examined the perceptions of 1,638 secondary IEP team members from almost 400 traditional educator-directed IEP meetings. Students knew the reasons for the meetings, knew what to do, and understood what was said at the meetings, but they also talked significantly less than all other participants, suggesting there is still a distance to go to achieve true student involvement. Special education teachers talked the most, and special educators and parents talked more about student interests than did the students. Indicative of the benefit of student participation, when students did attend their meetings, parents and general education teachers indicated that they understood the reasons for the meeting, felt more comfortable talking at the meeting, and understood more of what was said.

To verify these survey-based findings, Martin, Van Dycke, Greene, and colleagues (2006) observed 109 secondary teacher-directed IEP transition meetings using 10-second momentary time sampling to determine who talked in typical teacher-directed IEP meetings. As indicated in Figure 11.1, the results revealed that students talked during only 3% of the IEP meeting observations. Special education teachers directed the process, dominated the discussions, and appeared to have the greatest amount of satisfaction with the events and the issues discussed during the IEP meetings. Special educators spoke 51% of the time, family members spoke 15% of the time, general educators and administrators each spoke 9%, support person-nel spoke 6%, and multiple conversations occurred 5% of the meeting time. Stu-dent conversation at the meetings outranked only the category in which no one talked. Students reported knowing the reasons for the meetings and what they needed to do at the meetings significantly less than any other members of the IEP team. Over 70% of the participants indicated that a team member left early. Interestingly, almost 40% of the special education teachers and family members reported students talking a lot during the meeting. This perception starkly con-trasted with the results of direct observation. Perhaps this difference simply matched expectations held by the special education teachers and parents. Maybe parents and special education teachers equate attendance and only saying a few words with active participation.

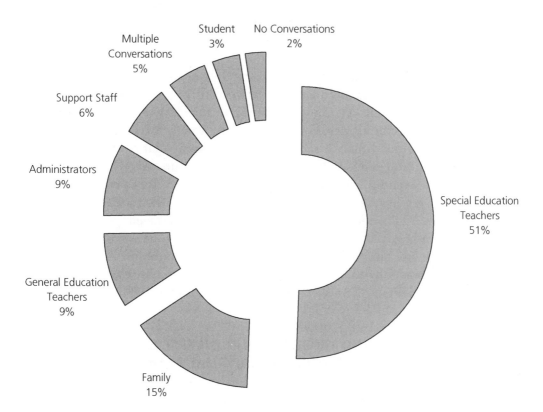

FIGURE 11.1. Percent of 10-second intervals that IEP team members talked during traditional educator-directed meetings. From Martin et al. (2006). Copyright 2006 by The Council for Excep-tional Children. Reprinted by permission.

After-meeting surveys by the IEP team verified the observations and indicated that special educators participated significantly more than any other participant. This participation included talking at the meetings, discussing students' needs and strengths, leading transition discussions, and helping with decision making. Other team members participated, but special education teachers dominated the meetings. Survey questions completed immediately after the IEP meetings indicated that transition planning received the lowest score of the four concepts discussed at the meetings. Students reported they minimally engaged in discussions about their postschool vision and only expressed their school and postschool interests during half of the observed meetings.

Van Dycke, Lovett, Greene, and Martin (2006) conducted a qualitative study of educator-directed IEP meetings, and several interesting themes emerged. The first theme, labeled "instant vision", was that special educators asked students to describe their interests and postschool vision with little to no preparation. From the student perspective, it was as if this request simply came out of the blue and, not surprisingly, students had little, if anything, to say or provided only brief responses to specific questions. The second theme, labeled "out of focus", was that meeting discussions occurred as if students were not present and that no student ownership of the IEP meeting or its discussion occurred. More than anyone else at the IEP table, parents had their discussion interrupted, typically by special education teachers as they guided the meeting back to the next issue on the IEP forms.

Students' lack of prior knowledge regarding the purpose of their transition IEP meeting, their lack of meaningful participation during the meetings, and their depressed feelings of comfort and respect during the meetings, provide evidence of a fundamental opportunity disadvantage. Martin, Van Dycke, Greene, and colleagues (2006) concluded that "it seems naïve to presume that students attending their transition IEP meetings will learn how to participate actively and lead this process through serendipity—yet this is precisely what current practice tends to expect" (p. 189). If we want students to participate actively, then we need explicitly to teach students skills and what to expect prior to their meetings and provide opportunities for engagement during the meetings. Unfortunately, schools do not typically engage students in their own educational planning process and, thus, miss a prime opportunity to increase student involvement and self-determination (Thoma, Held, & Sadler, 2002; Wehmeyer, Agran, & Hughes, 1998).

CULTURALLY AND LINGUISTICALLY DIVERSE STUDENTS, THEIR FAMILIES, AND EDUCATIONAL PLANNING

We have not discussed much concerning cultural and linguistic diversity with regard to promoting self-determination because, frankly, not much is known. A few studies (Frankland, Turnbull, Wehmeyer, & Blackmountain, 2004; Lee & Wehmeyer, 2004; Ohtake & Wehmeyer, 2004; Zhang, Wehmeyer, & Chen,

2005) have examined the relevance of the self-determination construct to non-Western cultures. By and large, these explorations suggest that promoting self-determination has relevance across cultures. The issue of cultural and linguistic diversity *has* been explored in the context of student involvement.

By the year 2040, over half the K–12 school population will be culturally and linguistically diverse students (Leake & Black, 2005; Archer, 2000; Sue, Bingham, Porshé-Burke, & Vasquez, 1999). Many culturally and linguistically diverse students come from family backgrounds that practice collective decision making, where plans are decided by the family's needs and interests (Black, Mrasek, & Ballinger, 2003). This contrasts with the individualist approach required during transition planning, when students need to tell their IEP team where *they* want to live, work, and continue their education after leaving school. The difference between school-based individualist planning and students' usual collective decision making poses unique issues that must be addressed during transition planning meetings.

The interrelationship among cultures, educational planning, and the IEP process influences postschool outcomes for students from culturally and linguistically diverse backgrounds (Leake, Black, & Roberts, 2004; Trainor, 2002). Postschool outcomes for culturally and linguistically diverse students with disabilities include lower rates of postsecondary education participation, lower rates of employment, and a lower percentage of workers earning more than minimum wage compared to students with disabilities identified as European American (Wagner, Newman, Cameto, & Levine, 2005).

Individualism and Collectivism

Many of the current educational planning practices teach students to set goals and plan for the future using practices that promote individualism (Zhang, 2005; Trainor, 2002; Valenzuela & Martin, 2005), meaning that students with disabilities are encouraged and expected to make their own decisions and attain their own goals. Self-determination practices that utilize personal decision making, self-evaluation, self-awareness, self-knowledge, and self-advocacy support an individualist perspective (Frankland et al., 2004). Students' family or group well-being and needs often shape the plans and goals of students from a collectivist background (Ewalt & Mokuau, 1995; Leake et al., 2004). Students from a collectivist background do not see themselves as separate from their tribe or family, which often defines who they are and what they will do.

Students typically move from one decision-making format to the other or meld individualist and collectivist characteristics for more effective interactions or to meet particular needs (Leake & Black, 2005). Individuals from both an individualist and collectivist perspective undergo "cultural frame-switching" from collectivist to individualist and back when expectations and situations demand (LaFromboise, Coleman, & Gerton, 1993). This ability to frame-switch enables students, especially those from a collectivist background, to interact successfully within an individualist school society and a collectivist home setting, but not all students easily accomplish this cultural frame-switching.

Educators need to understand the impact collectivist decision making has on the individualist-oriented educational planning process, but little empirical guidance exists on how. The intersection of the individual-goal-oriented school culture with collectivist family values may create a barrier that prevents students from engaging in their educational process. Planning for life after high school challenges most teenagers and their families. Students with disabilities and their families face an even more difficult time developing and achieving a postschool plan. Yet another layer of frustration and difficulty occurs for students with disabilities from culturally and linguistically diverse backgrounds and their families. For these teenagers, the educational planning process needs to frame-switch culturally. Success requires students, families, teachers, and significant others to develop common visions for the student's future. The educational planning team needs to attune students' goals, interests, skills, limits, and expectations for involvement to students' cultural traditions.

Cultural Reciprocity

Cultural reciprocity involves getting to know and understand each family and that teacher, student, and family cultural identity variables interact so that the planning team hears and respects all voices (Harry, Rueda, & Kalyanpur, 1999). In cultural reciprocity, awareness of different planning values can lead to families, students, and educators feeling empowered (Leake & Black, 2005). Sensitive use of cultural reciprocity will enable teachers and other professionals successfully to engage students from diverse cultures and from their families. Cultural reciprocity coupled with student-directed and other self-determination strategies will ensure better outcomes for these students (Valenzuela & Martin, 2005).

Cultural reciprocity provides a basis for mutual understanding between students with disabilities from culturally diverse backgrounds and educators from mainstream American culture (Kalyanpur & Harry, 2004). Many education professionals from mainstream American culture may not consider themselves as belonging to a particular culture and may not be aware of their individualistic values (Sue et al., 1999). Acknowledging cultural differences and then determining why they are important to the student and his or her family will lead to collaborative understanding all around (Harry et al., 1999).

Effective educational planning strategies typically involve identification of the student's and family's dreams and apprehensions about the future. The student's expressed interests, preferences, and strengths must also be considered. Yet, students with disabilities from culturally and linguistically diverse backgrounds continue to leave high school not achieving personal and culturally relevant outcomes. Perhaps the lack of student and family voices being heard at educational planning meetings contributes to this exodus.

PERSON-CENTERED PLANNING[1]

One means to ensure issues pertaining to cultural and linguistic diversity that affect student involvement are addressed is to engage in person-centered planning. In fact, many schools, agencies, and states now require the use of person-centered planning methods (Schwartz, Jacobson, & Holburn, 2000; Smull & Lakin, 2002). Person-centered planning creates a student's vision for the future, setting goals corresponding to that vision based on the student's interests and needs and developing and implementing a plan to attain those goals. To facilitate this process, the student and the most important people in his or her life meet to develop a vision of his or her future. Participants at the meeting set goals, develop a shared vision, and identify necessary supports to achieve these goals. Members of the group then commit to working to meet specific goals. Person-centered planning differs in at least three ways from traditional educator-directed planning (O'Brien & O'Brien, 2002). First, it reframes differences in performance away from diagnostic labels. Second, it involves family and friends in the planning process so that professionals do not dominate the process. Third, it focuses on students' capabilities rather than on their deficits.

Person-centered planning may be viewed as an outgrowth of the movement to include individuals with developmental disabilities fully in their communities (O'Brien & O'Brien, 2002). Person-centered planning alleviates the problem of focusing on student deficits by focusing on capacities and opportunities in people and the environment according to the student's vision of the future. Holburn (2002) stated that the goals of person-centered planning "reduce social isolation and segregation, establish friendships, increase opportunities to engage in preferred activities, develop competence, and promote respect" (p. 250). The planning process identifies barriers to attaining goals, then develops strategies to overcome the identified barriers.

Several formats for conducting person-centered planning exist, with similar components (Holburn, 2002; Schwartz et al., 2000; Smull, 1998) that include:

- Family, friends, and professionals participate voluntarily.
- The group values the views of everyone.
- The facilitator focuses the group and maps important aspects of the discussion for all members to see or access.
- The facilitator arranges discussion into themes such as history, preferences, dreams, and fears, which facilitate the development of the vision of a better future.
- Based on the vision, the group sets goals and identifies ways to attain the goals.

---

[1] We would like to acknowledge the assistance of Professor David L. Lovett at the University of Oklahoma for his contribution to this section.

- Individual members agree to take responsibility for meeting specific goals.
- The group continues to hold meetings to monitor progress toward achieving the goals and to make revisions to the plan as needed.

Holburn (2002) suggested that when person-centered planning fails, it does so because the team: (1) perceives the identified barriers to be too large, (2) lacks understanding of the procedures, (3) fails to support the process, (4) does not implement all person-centered planning components, (5) lacks an adequately trained facilitator, and (6) does not fully involve the student. Almost by definition, the process may not build a plan that fully reflects student interests, but rather interests made on behalf of the student by family, friends, and professionals (Wehmeyer, 2002).

A few qualitative studies reported that participants in person-centered planning had positive perceptions of the process (Holburn, Jacobson, Schwartz, Flory, & Vietze, 2004). Recent quantitative research studies also explored the dynamics and outcomes of the person-centered planning process.

Person-Centered Planning Research

Self-Determination and Instructional Efficiency

Cross, Cooke, Wood, and Test (1999) compared person-centered planning (i.e., MAPS—Making Action Plans) and the goal-choosing process from Marshall, Martin, Maxson, and Jerman's (1997) Choosing Employment Goals curriculum. Both methods increased student self-determination scores, but the Choosing Employment Goals approach had a greater overall effect on increasing student self-determination and did so with greater instructional efficiency.

Interest by Proxy Problems

Green, Middleton, and Reid (2000) compared student preferences identified through the person-centered planning process with the results of a hands-on, repeated-measure student preference assessment. The systematic preference assessment process discovered that the person with a disability studied did not prefer 33% of the items that the person-centered process identified. Martin, Woods, Sylvester, and Gardner (2005) compared vocational choices made by significant others to those systematically identified by students and adults with developmental disabilities. The choices made by parents, educators, and other caregivers on behalf of the person with a disability seldom matched the choices made by the individuals.

Lack of Student Voices

Miner and Bates (1997) compared a person-centered education planning meeting format to the typical educator-directed meeting. They found that students attended 91% of the person-centered planning meetings compared to 82% of traditional educator-directed IEP meetings. The researchers counted each time the student, parent, teacher, and other IEP team members talked for 15 seconds or more. There were statistically significant differences between the person-centered planning condition and the traditional educator-directed meetings. Parents became involved in statistically more discussions in the person-centered format than in the traditional educator-directed method. Interestingly, Miner and Bates (1997) did not mention the level of student participation during person-centered or educator-directed planning formats.

Positive Outcomes

Holburn and colleagues (2004) conducted a longitudinal study of person-centered planning outcomes compared to traditional interdisciplinary service planning outcomes. The results indicated that person-centered planning produced more positive outcomes compared to traditional staff-directed planning for adults with intellectual and developmental disabilities. The adults in the person-centered planning group left the institutional residences for community-based housing in statistically greater numbers and had improved quality of life. The researchers did not randomly assign participants to the control or treatment group and made no mention of the interactions of the adults with disabilities during the meetings.

Summary of Person-Centered Planning

What does all of this research tell us about person-centered planning? O'Brien (2002) indicated that he does not view person-centered planning "as the cause of change" (p. 263), but Holburn and colleagues (2004) found meaningful differences in long-term outcomes for adults who had person-centered planning meetings compared to those who had traditional staff-directed meetings. The voices of students and adults with disabilities at person-centered meetings do not seem to be present. Others decide on their behalf, and several studies demonstrate that proxy choice made by others has a good chance of not representing the true preferences of the student or adult with disabilities. As Wehmeyer (2002) indicated, "person-centered planning has always emphasized the role of significant others in planning, whereas student-directed planning processes have emphasized building student capacity to set or track goals or make decisions" (p. 57). Person-centered planning seems to invigorate teams to accomplish outcomes, but would the results be even more meaningful if student voices drove the process?

INCREASING STUDENT PARTICIPATION IN EDUCATIONAL PLANNING

Numerous opportunities for student engagement in the IEP process exist, but the traditional educator-directed meeting structure seldom encourages students to become engaged. To meet the intent of IDEA's transition reforms, at least three focal points are needed, mediated by students' skills and talents. First, students need to learn about the IEP process and their roles prior to going into their IEP meetings. If this is an inappropriate expectation for students with more severe disabilities, prior interest preference assessment should at least be done to ascertain student likes and dislikes (see Chapter 2). Second, adult team members need to learn how to facilitate student involvement. Third, school and adult participants need to establish the expectation that students become actively involved in their own meetings (Field, Hoffman, & Posch, 1997; Field, Martin, Miller, Ward, & Wehmeyer, 1998a, 1998b; Halpern, 1994; Martin & Marshall, 1995; Serna & Lau-Smith, 1995; Wehmeyer, Palmer, Agran, Mithaug, & Martin, 2000; Valenzuela & Martin, 2005).

Test, Aspel, and Everson (2006) noted that the educational planning process should facilitate student-informed choice making, student-directed transition planning, and student discovery of the skills needed in the postschool environment. Greene and Kochhar-Bryant (2003) suggested that the educational planning process needs to provide students the opportunity to answer five questions to the best of their ability:

1. What are my school, work, and community living interests and skills?
2. Where do I want to go to school, live, or work after leaving high school?
3. What courses will I take to prepare for the future?
4. What are my strengths, and what do I need to improve?
5. What do I need to learn to make my post–high school goals happen?

Recent research suggests that students become actively involved in their meetings when they are taught what to do, when they are provided the opportunity to become meaningfully involved in educational planning, and when adults *expect* student participation. Students are more likely to attend; express their interests, skills, and limits; and remember IEP goals after the meetings end if they were actively involved. Family members indicate greater satisfaction with the educational and transition plan when students actively participate and direct their own IEP meetings (Allen, Smith, Test, Flowers, & Wood, 2001; Martin, Van Dycke, Christensen, et al., 2006; Snyder, 2000, 2002; Snyder & Shapiro, 1997; Sweeney, 1997). The postschool vision sections of participating students' IEP documents included more comprehensive postschool transition statements than those of students who participated in teacher-directed educational planning meetings (Van Dycke, 2005). Transition-aged students who learn how to participate actively in their educational planning meetings and have the opportunity to do so also increase their overall level of self-determination skills (Martin, Van Dycke, Christensen, et al., 2006).

Mason, Field, and Sawilowsky (2004) found that students and teachers value student involvement in the IEP meeting but that logistical challenges make this difficult: "Chief among these is finding the time necessary for adequate student preparation. With the trend away from pull-out resource rooms toward inclusion in the general classroom, teachers are finding it difficult to schedule time to prepare students for IEP meetings" (p. 188). But this time must be found. Students need time to think about what they want to say and time to prepare how they will add their voice to the educational planning meeting discussions. Student-directed educational practice demands student engagement in the educational planning process.

The Self-Directed IEP

A growing number of instructional programs exist for educators to teach students how to become actively involved in their IEP meetings (see Table 11.1). The Self-Directed IEP (Martin, Marshall, Maxson, & Jerman, 1997) systematically teaches students 11 steps to become engaged in their own IEP meetings. The instructional program uses video modeling, systematic instruction, student activities, and role playing to teach participation and IEP leadership skills. Numerous studies by different research groups across the United States have demonstrated the effectiveness of the Self-Directed IEP, so it can now be considered an evidence-based practice to increase student participation in IEP meetings. Although it was designed for students who have at least some reading and writing skills, teachers often adapt the material for use by students who do not read or write.

Impact of the Self-Directed IEP

Sweeney (1997) taught the Self-Directed IEP to a group of students, including some who required support for their cognitive disabilities. She found that the students with cognitive disabilities who received Self-Directed IEP instruction attended 100% of their meetings, compared to 22% of those in the teacher-directed IEP meeting condition, and that 83% of the students reported knowing two goals after the

TABLE 11.1. Instructional Materials That Have at Least Some Effectiveness Data with Students with Intellectual and Developmental Disabilities and Are Readily Available for Teachers to Teach Students IEP Meeting-Participation Skills

Program	Authors	Publisher	Demonstrated effectiveness
Self-Directed IEP	Martin, Marshall, Maxson, & Jerman, 1997	Sopris West	Strong
Whose Future Is It Anyway?	Wehmeyer et al., 2004	Beach Center on Disability	Moderate
NEXT S.T.E.P.	Halpern et al., 1997	Pro-Ed	Some
TAKE CHARGE for the Future	Powers et al., 2001	Portland State University	Some
Student-Led IEPs	McGahee, Mason, Wallace, & Jones, 2001	CEC	Limited

meeting, compared to 11% of students in the teacher-directed IEP condition. Snyder (2002) used the Self-Directed IEP to teach five students dually diagnosed with mental retardation and emotional problems to become actively engaged in their IEP meetings. Allen and colleagues (2001) taught students with mental retardation a modified version of the Self-Directed IEP to state the purpose of the meeting, introduce everyone, review past goals and performance, and close the meeting.

Martin, Van Dycke, Christensen, and colleagues (2006) conducted a large-group experimental study with 130 secondary-aged students and found that the Self-Directed IEP instructional program enabled students with disabilities to: (1) start and lead significantly more IEP meetings, (2) talk significantly more during the meetings, (3) engage in significantly more IEP meeting leadership steps, and (4) report in postmeeting surveys significantly higher positive perceptions of their IEP meetings. Students and adults also reported significantly higher ratings of transition discussions in the postmeeting surveys. No significant time difference was found between the student-directed meetings and traditional educator-directed meetings. ChoiceMaker Self-Determination Assessment (Martin & Marshall, 1995) found that Self-Directed IEP instruction significantly increased opportunities to learn self-determination skills. The assessment also showed the strong effect that Self-Directed IEP instruction had on student involvement and goal attainment self-determination measures.

Van Dycke (2005) found that the actual IEP documents of students in the Martin, Van Dycke, Christensen, and colleagues (2006) study who received Self-Directed IEP instruction had more comprehensive postschool transition statements. The students in this study included those with learning disabilities, emotional problems, intellectual disabilities, autism, and other health impairments. Martin, Van Dycke, Christensen, and colleagues (2006) did not present results by severity of support need or by disability category. They also compared students with intellectual disabilities and autism who received Self-Directed IEP instruction (nine students) to those who participated in typical teacher-directed IEP meetings (seven students) to determine the percent of the time students talked at their IEP meetings and the percent of leadership steps they engaged in with and without prompting. Figure 11.2 presents the percent of time students and other team members talked at the IEP meetings. Students with intellectual disabilities and autism in the teacher-directed meetings talked 4% of the time, while students with intellectual disabilities and autism who received Self-Directed IEP instruction talked 11% of the time. Special education teachers and parents talked less when students became more engaged. When students increased their participation, so did general educators. The general educators increased their talking four times and the incidence of multiple conversations and periods of no conversations across all team members decreased.

As depicted in Figure 11.3, students with intellectual disabilities and autism who received Self-Directed IEP instruction (eight students) engaged in more IEP meeting leadership steps than students who participated in teacher-directed IEP

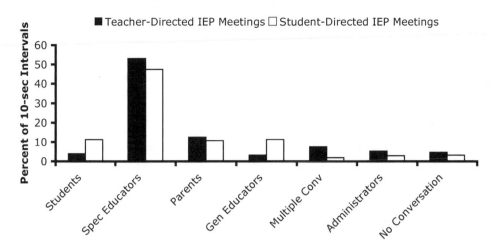

FIGURE 11.2. Percent of 10-second intervals that IEP team members comparing students who received Self-Directed IEP instruction to those who participated in teacher-directed IEP meetings.

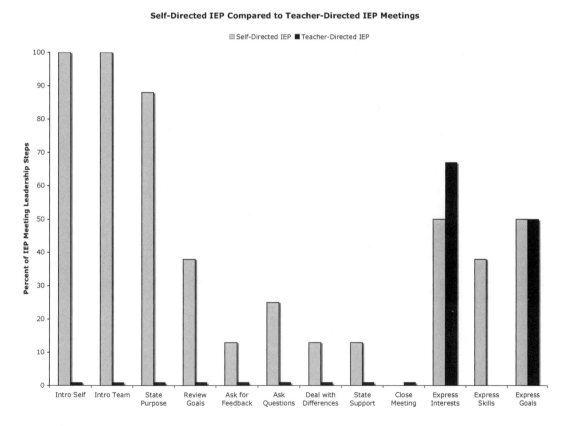

FIGURE 11.3. Percent completed of IEP leadership steps by students with intellectual disabilities and autism who received Self-Directed IEP instruction compared to those who participated in teacher-directed IEP meetings.

meetings (six students). All of the students who received Self-Directed IEP instruction introduced themselves and their IEP team, and most stated the purpose of the meeting. Half the students expressed their interests and goals, and up to one third of the students reviewed past goals and their performance on those goals, asked for feedback, asked questions, stated support needs, and expressed their skills and/or limits. Students engaged in 40% of these leadership steps independently (without teacher prompting). Students in the teacher-directed meetings only discussed their interests about two-thirds of the time and engaged in conversations about their goals about half the time. Students in the teacher-directed meeting condition engaged in 39% of these two steps independently (without teacher prompting).

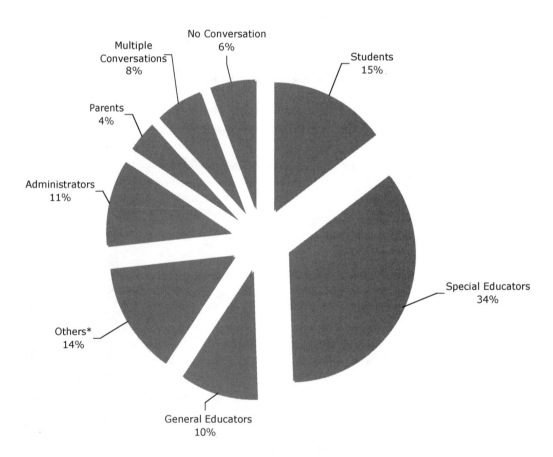

Percent of Time Students Blind and with MR or Autism Talked at Their IEP Meetings

FIGURE 11.4. Percent of 10-second intervals that IEP team members talked where students received Self-Directed IEP instruction and IEP team received brief instruction on how to facilitate student involvement. *Other members included speech therapists, assistive technology teachers, vocational rehab counselors, orientation and mobility teachers, and a living skill coach.

Wu, Martin, and Isabell (2006) conducted a study that examined the use of the Self-Directed IEP by teachers at the Oklahoma School for the Blind, who taught 33 secondary students using the Self-Directed IEP. As depicted in Figure 11.4, these students talked an average of 15% of the time, special education teachers 34% of the time, and general educators 10% of the time, with the remaining team members talking 4% to 14% of the time. No conversations and multiple conversations accounted for 12% of the observations.

Whose Future Is It Anyway?

Whose Future Is It Anyway? (Wehmeyer et al., 2004) is another student-involvement approach with efficacy data pertaining to students with intellectual and developmental disabilities. It consists of 36 sessions introducing students to the concept of transition and transition planning and enabling students to self-direct instruction related to (1) self- and disability awareness, (2) making decisions about transition-related outcomes, (3) identifying and securing community resources to support transition services, (4) writing and evaluating transition goals and objectives, (5) communicating effectively in small groups, and (6) developing skills to become an effective team member, leader, or self-advocate.

The materials are student-directed in that they are written for students as end-users. The level of support needed by students to complete activities varies a great deal. Some students with difficulty reading or writing need one-on-one support to progress through the materials; others can complete the process independently. The materials make every effort to ensure that students retain this control while at the same time receiving the support they need to succeed.

Section 1 (titled Getting to Know You) introduces the concept of transition and educational planning, provides information about transition requirements in IDEA, and enables students to identify who has attended past planning meetings, who is required to be present at meetings, and who they want involved in their planning process. Later, they are introduced to four transition outcome areas (employment, community living, postsecondary education, and recreation and leisure). Activities throughout the process focus on these transition outcome areas. The remainder of the sessions in this first section discuss the topic of disability and disability awareness. Students identify their unique characteristics, including their abilities and interests, then identify unique learning needs related to their disability; finally, students identify their unique learning needs *resulting* from their disability.

In the second section (Making Decisions), students learn a simple problem-solving process by working through each step to make a decision about a potential living arrangement, then apply the process to make decisions about the three other transition outcome areas. The third section (How to Get What You Need, Sec. 101) enables students to locate community resources identified in previous planning meetings that are intended to provide supports in each of the transition outcome areas. The fourth section (Goals, Objectives and the Future) enables learners to apply a set of rules to identify transition-related goals and objectives that are currently on their IEP or transition-planning form, evaluate these goals based on their transition interests and abilities, and develop additional goals to take to their next planning meeting. Students learn what goals and objectives are, how they should be written, and ways to track their progress.

The fifth section (Communicating) introduces effective communication strategies for small-group situations, like the transition-planning meetings. Students work through sessions that introduce different types of communication (verbal, body language, etc.) and how to interpret these communicative behaviors, the differences between aggressive and assertive communication, how to negotiate and compromise effectively, when to use persuasion, and other skills that will enable them to be more effective communicators during transition-planning meetings. The final session (Thank You, Honorable Chairperson) enables students to learn types and purposes of meetings, steps to holding effective meetings, and roles of the meeting chairperson and team members. Students are encouraged to work with school personnel to take a meaningful role in planning for and participating in the meeting.

Students are encouraged to work on one session per week during the weeks between their previous transition-planning meeting and the next scheduled meeting. The final two sessions review the previous sessions and provide a refresher for students as they head into their planning meeting. These materials have been field tested and validated for use with students with cognitive disabilities (Wehmeyer & Lawrence, 1995, in press) and shown to affect student self-determination, self-efficacy for educational planning, and student involvement.

Next S.T.E.P.: Student Transition and Educational Planning

A third student-directed transition-planning program is the Next S.T.E.P curriculum (Halpern et al., 1997). The curriculum uses video and print materials developed for specific audiences (students, teachers, family members) to help students become motivated to engage in transition planning, self-evaluate transition needs, identify and select transition goals and activities, assume responsibility for conducting their own transition-planning meeting, and monitor the implementation of their transition plans.

The curriculum consists of 16 lessons, clustered into four instructional units, designed to be delivered in a 50-minute class period. These lessons include teacher and student materials, videos, guidelines for involving parents and family members and a process for tracking student progress. Unit 1 (Getting Started) introduces and overviews transition planning to enable students to understand the transition-planning process and to motivate them to participate. Unit 2 (Self-Exploration and Self-Evaluation) includes six lessons that focus on student self-evaluation. Students work through activities that identify unique interests, strengths, and weaknesses in various adult-outcome-oriented areas. At the end of this unit, students complete the student form of the Transition Skills Inventory, a 72-item rating instrument assessing how well the student is doing in four transition areas: (1) personal life, (2) jobs, (3) education and training, and (4) living on one's own. The student's self-evaluation of these areas is combined with similar evaluations by his or her teacher and a family member to form a basis for future transition-planning activities. Students are encouraged to discuss differences of opinion between the teacher or family member evaluations and their self-evaluation and to resolve these discrepancies either before or during the transition-planning meeting.

Unit 3 (Developing Goals and Activities) includes five lessons regarding transition goal identification in the four areas of the Transition Skills Inventory. Students identify their hopes and dreams, then select from a range of potential goals in each area, narrowing the total set of transition goals to four or five goals that they prefer. In addition, students choose activities that will help them pursue the goals they have selected. Unit 4 (Putting a Plan into Place) includes three lessons preparing students for their transition-planning meeting. The lessons emphasize the implementation of their plan and work with students to ensure that they monitor their progress and, if necessary, make adjustments. Zhang (2001) examined the efficacy of the Next S.T.E.P. materials and found implementation significantly affected student self-determination.

TAKE CHARGE for the Future

TAKE CHARGE for the Future (Powers, Sowers, et al., 1996) is a student-directed, collaborative model to promote student involvement in educational and transition planning. The model is an adaptation of a validated approach, referred to as TAKE CHARGE, to promote the self-determination of youth with and without disabilities (Powers et al., 1998). TAKE CHARGE uses four components or strategies to promote adolescent development of self-determination: skill facilitation, mentoring, peer support, and parent support. For example, TAKE CHARGE introduces youth to three major skill areas needed to take charge in one's life: achievement skills, partnership skills, and coping skills. Youth involved in the TAKE CHARGE process are matched with successful adults of the same sex who experience similar challenges and share common interests and are involved in peer support activities throughout (Powers, Sowers, et al., 1996). Parental support is provided via information and technical assistance and written materials.

TAKE CHARGE uses the same set of core strategies to enable learners with disabilities to participate in their planning meeting. Students are provided self-help materials and coaching to identify their transition goals, to organize and conduct transition-planning meetings, and to achieve their goals through the application of problem-solving, self-regulation, and partnership management strategies. Concurrently, youth participate in self-selected mentorship and peer support activities to increase their transition-focused knowledge and skills. Their parents are also provided with information and support to promote their capacities to encourage their sons' or daughters' active involvement in transition planning. Powers, Turner, Matuszewski, Wilson, and Phillips (2001) conducted a control-group study and found that the TAKE CHARGE materials positively affected student involvement.

Student-Led IEPs: A Guide for Student Involvement

McGahee, Mason, Wallace, and Jones (2001) developed a guide to student-led IEPs (available online at www.nichcy.org/stuguid.asp) that introduces students to the IEP process, the purpose of an IEP, and suggestions for writing an IEP. Mason, McGahee-Kovac, Johnson, and Stillerman (2002) showed that students who used this process knew more about their IEP and showed enhanced self-confidence and self-advocacy.

SUMMARY

The research suggests that as we teach students the skills to become more involved in their IEP meetings, provide opportunities for students to participate, and teach other IEP team members how to facilitate student involvement, students *do* actively participate. Active involvement in educational planning teaches public speaking, self-advocacy, goal setting, self-evaluation, and adjustment of goals and strategies. Equally important, as students increase their level of participation, other IEP team members become more involved in the meeting, IEP team members report feeling better about their meetings, and students increase their overall level of self-determination skills.

Person-centered planning brings new voices to the educational planning process, but not necessarily the voices of students. Our field also needs to examine the long-term impact of increased student involvement on school performance, family involvement, and postschool outcomes. Some research suggests that increasing student involvement in educational planning meetings increases students' level of self-determination. We need to create as many opportunities as possible for students to learn and practice their self-determination skills, including becoming involved in their educational meetings.

References

Abery, B., Smith, J., Sharpe, M. N., & Chelberg, G. (1995). From the editors. *IMPACT: Feature Issue on Leadership by Persons with Disabilities, 8*(3), 1.

Agran, M. (Ed.). (1997). *Student-directed learning: Teaching self-determination skills.* Pacific Grove, CA: Brooks/Cole.

Agran, M., Blanchard, C., Hughes, C., & Wehmeyer, M. L. (2002). Increasing the problem-solving skills of students with severe disabilities participating in general education. *Remedial and Special Education, 23,* 279–288.

Agran, M., Blanchard, C., & Wehmeyer, M. L. (2000). Promoting transition goals and self-determination through student-directed learning: The self-determined learning model of instruction. *Education and Training in Mental Retardation and Developmental Disabilities, 35,* 351–364.

Agran, M., Blanchard, C., Wehmeyer, M., & Hughes, C. (2001). Teaching students to self-regulate their behavior: The differential effects of students vs. teacher-delivered reinforcement. *Research in Developmental Disabilities, 22,* 319–332.

Agran, M., Cain, H. M., & Cavin, M. D. (2002). Enhancing the involvement of rehabilitation counselors in the transition process. *Career Development for Exceptional Individuals, 25,* 141–155.

Agran, M., Cavin, M., Wehmeyer, M. L., & Palmer, S. (2006). Participation of students with severe disabilities in the general curriculum: The effects of the self-determined learning model of instruction. *Research and Practice in Severe Disabilities, 31,* 230–241.

Agran, M., Fodor-Davis, J., & Moore, S. (1986). The effects of self-instructional training on job-task sequencing: Suggesting a problem-solving strategy. *Education and Training of the Mentally Retarded, 21,* 273–281.

Agran, M., Fodor-Davis, J., Moore, S., & Deer, M. (1989). The application of a self-management program on instruction-following skills. *Journal of the Association for Persons with Severe Handicaps, 14,* 147–154.

Agran, M., & Hughes, C. (1997). Problem solving. In M. Agran (Ed.), *Student-directed learning: Teaching self-determination skills* (pp. 171–198). Pacific Grove, CA: Brooks/Cole.

Agran, M., & Hughes, C. (2005). Introduction to the special issue on self-determination: How far have we come? *Research and Practice for Persons with Severe Disabilities, 30*, 105–107.

Agran, M., Hughes, C., & Washington, B. (2006). *Student-centered educational programming: What do students say?* Manuscript in preparation.

Agran, M., King-Sears, M., Wehmeyer, M. L., & Copeland, S. (2003). *Teacher's guide to inclusive practice: Student-directed learning.* Baltimore: Brookes.

Agran, M., & Martin, J. E. (1987). Applying a technology of self-control in community environments for individuals who are mentally retarded. In M. Hersen, R. M. Eisler, & P. M. Miller (Eds.), *Progress in behavior modification* (Vol. 21, pp. 108–151). Newbury Park, CA: Sage.

Agran, M., & Moore, S. (1994). *How to teach self-instruction job skills.* Washington, DC: American Association on Mental Retardation.

Agran, M., Salzberg, C. L., & Stowitschek, J. J. (1987). An analysis of the effects of a social skills training program using self-instructions on the acquisition and generalization of two social behaviors in a working setting. *Journal of the Association for Persons with Severe Handicaps, 12*, 131–139.

Agran, M., Sinclair, T., Alper, S., Cavin, M. L., Wehmeyer, M., & Hughes, C. (2005). Using self-monitoring to increase following-direction skills of students with moderate to severe disabilities in general education. *Education and Training in Developmental Disabilities, 40*, 3–13.

Algozzine, B., Browder, D., Karvonen, M., Test, D. W., & Wood, W. M. (2001). Effects of intervention to promote self-determination for individuals with disabilities. *Review of Educational Research, 71*, 219–277.

Allen, S. K., Smith, A. C., Test, D. W., Flowers, C., & Wood, W. M. (2001). The effects of Self-Directed IEP on student participation in IEP meetings. *Career Development for Exceptional Individuals, 24*, 107–120.

American Heritage dictionary of the English language, The. (1992). New York: Houghton Mifflin.

Ames, C. (1992). Achievement goals and the classroom motivational climate. In D. H. Schunk & J. L. Meece (Eds.), *Student perceptions in the classroom* (pp. 327–348). Hillsdale, NJ: Erlbaum.

Archer, J. (2000). Competition is fierce for minority teachers. *Education Week, 19*, 32–33.

Baer, D. M. (1984). Does research on self-control need more control? *Analysis and Intervention in Developmental Disabilities, 4*, 211–218.

Balcazar, F. E., Keys, C. B., & Garate-Serafini, J. (1995). Learning to recruit assistance to attain transition goals: A program for adjudicated youth with disabilities. *Remedial and Special Education, 16*, 237–246.

Balcazar, F. E., Seekins, T., Fawcett, S. B., and Hopkins, B. L. (1990). Empowering people with physical disabilities through advocacy skills training. *American Journal of Community Psychology, 18*, 281–296.

Bambara, L. M. (2004). Fostering choice-making skills: We've come a long way but still have a long way to go. *Research and Practice for Persons with Severe Disabilities, 29*, 169–171.

Bambara, L. M., & Ager, C. (1992). Using self-scheduling to promote self-directed leisure activity in home community settings. *Journal of the Association for Persons with Severe Handicaps, 17*, 67–76.

Bambara, L. M., & Gomez, O. N. (2001). Using a self-instructional training package to teach complex problem-solving skills to adults with moderate and severe disabilities. *Education and Training in Mental Retardation and Developmental Disabilities, 36,* 386–400.

Bandura, A. (1969). *Principles of behavior modification.* New York: Holt, Rinehart and Winston.

Bandura, A. (1997). *Self-efficacy: The exercise of control.* New York: Freeman.

Barling, J., & Patz, M. (1980). Differences following self- and external reinforcement as a function of locus of control and age: A social learning analysis. *Personality and Individual Differences, 1,* 79–85.

Basquill, M. F., Nezu, C. M., Nezu, A. M., & Klein, T. L. (2004). Agression-related hostility bias and social problem-solving deficits in adult males with mental retardation. *American Journal of Mental Retardation, 109,* 255–263.

Bates, P. (1980). The effectiveness of interpersonal skills training on the social skill acquisition of moderately and mildly retarded adults. *Journal of Applied Behavior Analysis, 13,* 237–248.

Battle, D. A., Dickens-Wright, L. L., & Murphy, S. C. (1998). How to empower adolescents: Guidelines for effective self-advocacy. *Teaching Exceptional Children, 30,* 28–33.

Benjamin, C. (1996a). *Problem solving in school.* Upper Saddle River, NJ: Globe Fearon Educational Publisher.

Benjamin, C. (1996b). *Problem solving on the job.* Upper Saddle River, NJ: Globe Fearon Educational Publisher.

Berg, W. K., Wacker, D. P., & Flynn, T. H. (1990). Teaching generalization and maintenance of work behavior. In F. R. Rusch (Ed.), *Supported employment: Models, methods, and issues* (pp. 145–160). Sycamore, IL: Sycamore.

Beyth-Marom, R., Fischhoff, B., Jacobs Quadrel, M., & Furby, L. (1991). Teaching decision making to adolescents: A critical review. In J. Baron & R. V. Brown (Eds.), *Teaching decision making to adolescents* (pp. 19–59). Hillsdale, NJ: Erlbaum.

Black, R. S., Mrasek, K. D., & Ballinger, R. (2003). Individualist and collectivist values in transition planning for culturally diverse students with special needs. *Journal for Vocational Special Needs Education, 25,* 20–29.

Bornstein, P. H., Bach, P. J., McFall, M. E., Friman, P. C., & Lyons, P. D. (1980). Application of a social skills training program in the modification of interpersonal deficits among retarded adults: A clinical replication. *Journal of Applied Behavior Analysis, 13,* 171–176.

Branham, R. S., Collins, B. C., Schuster, J. W., & Kleinert, H. (1999). Teaching community skills to students with moderate disabilities: Comparing combined techniques of classroom simulation, videotape modeling, and community-based instruction. *Education and Training in Mental Retardation and Developmental Disabilities, 34,* 170–181.

Bransford, J. D., & Stein, B. S. (1993). *The IDEAL problem solver* (2nd ed.). New York: Freeman.

Bregman, S. (1984). Assertiveness training for mentally retarded adults. *Mental Retardation, 22,* 12–16.

Brim, G. (1992). *Ambition: How we manage success and failure throughout our lives.* New York: Basic Books.

Brinton, B., & Fujiki, M. (1993). Communication skills and community integration in adults with mild to moderate retardation. *Topics in Language Disorders, 13*(3), 9–19.

Browder, D. M., Cooper, K. J., & Lim, L. (1998). Teaching adults with severe disabilities to express their choice of settings for leisure activities. *Education and Training in Mental Retardation and Developmental Disabilities, 33,* 228–238.

Browder, D. M., & Minarovic, T. J. (2000). Utilizing sight words in self-instruction training for employees with moderate mental retardation in competitive jobs. *Education and Training in Mental Retardation and Developmental Disabilities, 35,* 78–89.

Brown, F., Belz, P., Corsi, L., & Wenig, B. (1993). Choice and diversity for people with severe disabilities. *Education and Training in Mental Retardation, 28,* 318–326.

Brown, F., Gothelf, C. R., Guess, D., & Lehr, D. (1998). Self-determination for individuals with the most severe disabilities: Moving beyond chimeras. *Journal of the Association for Persons with Severe Handicaps, 23,* 17–26.

Browning, P., & Nave, G. (1993). Teaching social problem solving to learners with mild disabilities. *Education and Training in Mental Retardation, 28,* 309–317.

Bullock, C. C., & Mahon, M. J. (1992). Decision making in leisure: Empowerment for people with mental retardation. *Journal of Physical Education, Recreation and Dance, 63*(8), 36–40.

Cameto, R., Levine, P., and Wagner, M. (2004). *Transition planning for students with disabilities. A special topic report of findings from the National Longitudinal Transition Study-2 (NLTS2).* Menlo Park, CA: SRI International.

Cannella, H. I., O'Reilly, M. F., & Lancioni, G. E. (2005). Choice and preference assessment research with people with severe to profound developmental disabilities: A review of the literature. *Research in Developmental Disabilities, 26,* 1–15.

Carr, J. E., Nicolson, A. C., & Higbee, T. S. (2000). Evaluation of a brief multiple-stimulus preference assessment in a naturalistic content. *Journal of Applied Behavior Analysis, 33,* 353–357.

Castles, E. E., & Glass, C. R. (1986). Training in social and interpersonal problem-solving skills for mildly and moderately mentally retarded adults. *American Journal of Mental Deficiency, 91,* 35–42.

Castro, L., & Rachline, H. (1980). Self-reward, self-monitoring, and self-punishment as feedback in weight control. *Behavior Therapy, 11,* 38–48.

Cea, C. D., & Fisher, C. B. (2003). Health-care decisions made by adults with mental retardation. *Mental Retardation, 41,* 78–87.

Center for Universal Design. (1997). *Principles of universal design.* Raleigh, NC: The Center for Universal Design, North Carolina State University.

Coleman, M., Wheeler, L., & Webber, J. (1993). Research on interpersonal problem-solving training: A review. *Remedial and Special Education, 14,* 25–37.

Collet-Klingenberg, L., & Chadsey-Rusch, J. (1991). Using a cognitive-process approach to teach social skills. *Education and Training in Mental Retardation, 26,* 258–270.

Columbus, M. A., & Mithaug, D. E. (2003). The effects of self-regulation problem-solving instruction on the self-determination of secondary students with disabilities. In D. E. Mithaug, D. K. Mithaug, M. Agran, J. E. Martin, & M. L. Wehmeyer (Eds.), *Self-determined learning theory: Construction, verification, and evaluation* (pp. 172–187). Mahwah, NJ: Erlbaum.

Cooper, K. J., & Browder, D. M. (1998). Enhancing choice and participation for adults with severe disabilities in community-based instruction. *Journal of the Association for Persons with Severe Handicaps, 23,* 252–260.

Cooper, L. J., Wacker, D. P., Thursby, D., Plagmann, L. A., Harding, J., Millard, T., et al. (1992). Analysis of the effects of task preferences, task demands, and adult attention on child behavior in outpatient and classroom settings. *Journal of Applied Behavior Analysis, 25,* 823–840.

Copeland, S. R., & Hughes, C. (2002). Effects of goal setting on task performance of persons with mental retardation. *Education and Training in Mental Retardation and Developmental Disabilities, 37*, 40–54.

Copeland, S. R., Hughes, C., Agran, M., Wehmeyer, M. L., & Fowler, S. E. (2002). An intervention package to support high school students with mental retardation in general education classrooms. *American Journal of Mental Retardation, 107*, 32–45.

Coyle, C., & Cole, P. (2004). A videotaped self-modeling and self-monitoring treatment program to decrease off-task behaviour in children with autism. *Journal of Intellectual and Developmental Disabilities, 29*, 3–16.

Cross, T., Cooke, N. L., Wood, W. M., & Test, D. W. (1999). Comparison of the effects of MAPS and ChoiceMaker on student self-determination skills. *Education and Training in Mental Retardation and Developmental Disabilities, 34*, 499–510.

Crouch, K. P., Rusch, F. R., & Karlan, G. R. (1984). Competitive employment utilizing the correspondence training paradigm to enhance productivity. *Education and Training of the Mentally Retarded, 19*, 268–275.

Csikszentmilhalyi, M. (1990). *Flow: The psychology of optimal experience.* New York: Harper & Row.

Dalton, T., Martella, R. C., & Marchand-Martella, N. E. (1999). The effects of a self-management program in reducing off-task behavior. *Journal of Behavioral Education, 9*, 157–176.

Dattilo, J. (1986). Computerized assessment of preference for severely handicapped individuals. *Journal of Applied Behavior Analysis, 19*, 445–448.

Datillo, J., & Hoge, G. (1999). Effects of a leisure education program on youth with mental retardation. *Education and Training in Mental Retardation and Developmental Disabilities, 34*, 20–34.

Dattilo, J., & Mirenda, P. (1987). An application of a leisure preference assessment protocol for persons with severe handicaps. *Journal of the Association for Persons with Severe Handicaps, 12*, 306–311.

Davies, D. K., Stock, S., & Wehmeyer, M. L. (2001). Enhancing independent Internet access for individuals with mental retardation through the use of a specialized web browser: A pilot study. *Education and Training in Mental Retardation and Developmental Disabilities, 36*, 107–113.

Davies, D. K., Stock, S., & Wehmeyer, M. L. (2002a). Enhancing independent task performance for individuals with mental retardation through use of a handheld self-directed visual and audio prompting system. *Education and Training in Mental Retardation and Developmental Disabilities, 37*, 209–218.

Davies, D. K., Stock, S., & Wehmeyer, M. L. (2002b). Enhancing independent time-management skills of individuals with mental retardation using a palmtop personal computer. *Mental Retardation, 40*, 358–365.

Davies, D. K., Stock, S., & Wehmeyer, M. L. (2003a). Application of computer simulation to teach ATM access to individuals with intellectual disabilities. *Education and Training in Developmental Disabilities, 38*, 451–456.

Davies, D. K., Stock, S., & Wehmeyer, M. L. (2003b). A palmtop computer-based intelligent aid for individuals with intellectual disabilities to increase independent decision making. *Research and Practice for Persons with Severe Disabilities, 28*, 182–193.

Davies, D. K., Stock, S., & Wehmeyer, M. L. (2004). Computer-mediated, self-directed computer training and skill assessment for individuals with mental retardation. *Journal of Physical and Developmental Disabilities, 16*, 95–105.

Deci, E. L. (1975). *Intrinsic motivation.* New York: Plenum Press.

Deci, E. L. (1992). The relation of interest to the motivation of behavior: A self-determination theory perspective. In K. A. Renninger, S. Hidi, & A. Krapp (Eds.), *The role of interest in learning and development* (pp. 43–70). Hillsdale, NJ: Erlbaum.

Deci, E. L., & Chandler, C. L. (1986). The importance of motivation for the future of the LD field. *Journal of Learning Disabilities, 19,* 587–594.

Deci, E. L., & Ryan, R. (1985). *Intrinsic motivation and self-determination in human behavior.* New York: Plenum Press.

Deci, E. L., & Ryan, R. (2003). *The handbook of self-determination research.* Rochester, NY: University of Rochester Press.

Dibley, S., & Lim, L. (1999). Providing choice making opportunities within and between daily school routines. *Journal of Behavioral Education, 9,* 117–132.

Dickerson, E. A., & Creedon, C. F. (1981). Self-selection of standards by children: The relative effectiveness of pupil-selected and teacher-selected standards of performance. *Journal of Applied Behavior Analysis, 14,* 423–433.

Doll, E., Sands, D., Wehmeyer, M. L., & Palmer, S. (1996). Promoting the development and acquisition of self-determined behavior. In D. J. Sands & M. L. Wehmeyer (Eds.), *Self-determination across the life span: Independence and choice for people with disabilities* (pp. 65–90). Baltimore: Brookes.

Domingo, R. A., Barrow, M. B., & Amato, J. (1998). Excercise of linguistic control by speakers in an adult day treatment program. *Mental Retardation, 36,* 293–302.

Dweck, C. S. (1986). Motivational processes affecting learning. *American Psychologist, 41,* 1040–1048.

D'Zurilla, T. J. (1986). *Problem-solving therapy.* New York: Springer.

D'Zurilla, T. J., & Goldfried, M. R. (1971). Problem solving and behavior modification. *Journal of Abnormal Psychology, 78,* 107–126.

Eder, R. (1990). Uncovering young children's psychological selves: Individual and developmental differences. *Child Development, 61,* 849–863.

Edgerton, R. B. (1988). Aging in the community: A matter of choice. *American Journal of Mental Retardation, 92,* 331–335.

Elias, M. J., Branden-Muller, L. R., & Sayette, M. A. (1991). Teaching the foundations of social decision making and problem solving in the elementary school. In J. Baron & R. V. Brown (Eds.), *Teaching decision making to adolescents* (pp. 161–184). Hillsboro, NJ: Erlbaum.

Ellis, N. R., Woodley-Zanthos, P., Dulaney, C. L., & Palmer, R. L. (1989). Automatic effortful processing and cognitive inertia in persons with mental retardation. *American Journal of Mental Retardation, 93,* 412–423.

Ewalt, P. L., & Mokuau, N. (1995). Self-determination from a Pacific perspective. *Social Work, 40,* 168–175.

Fantuzzo, J. W., & Clement, P. W. (1981). Generalization of the effects of teacher- and self-administered token reinforcers to nontreated students. *Journal of Applied Behavior Analysis, 14,* 435–447.

Faw, G. D., Davis, P. K., & Peck, C. (1996). Increasing self-determination: Teaching people with mental retardation to evaluate residential options. *Journal of Applied Behavior Analysis, 29,* 173–188.

Ferretti, R. P., & Butterfield, E. C. (1989). Intelligence as a correlate of children's problem-solving. *American Journal of Mental Retardation, 93,* 424–433.

Ferretti, R. P., & Cavalier, A. R. (1991). Constraints on the problem solving of persons with mental retardation. In N. W. Bray (Ed.), *International review of research in mental retardation* (Vol. 17, pp. 153–192). San Diego, CA: Academic Press.

Feuerstein, R. (1979). *The dynamic assessment of retarded performers*. Baltimore: University Park Press.

Feuerstein, R. (1980). *Instrumental enrichment*. Baltimore: University Park Press.

Field, S., Hoffman, A., & Posch, M. (1997). Self-determination during adolescence: A developmental perspective. *Remedial and Special Education, 18*(5), 285–293.

Field, S., Martin, J. E., Miller, R. J., Ward, M., & Wehmeyer, M. L. (1998a). *A practical guide for teaching self-determination*. Reston, VA: Council for Exceptional Children.

Field, S., Martin, J. E., Miller, R., Ward, M., & Wehmeyer, M. L. (1998b). Self-determination for persons with disabilities: A position statement of the division on career development and transition. *Career Development for Exceptional Individuals, 21*, 113–128.

Foshay, J., & Ludlow, B. (2006). Implementing computer-mediated supports and assistive technology. In M. L. Wehmeyer & M. Agran (Eds.), *Mental retardation and intellectual disabilities: Teaching students using innovative and research-based strategies* (pp. 101–124). Boston: Pearson.

Foster-Johnson, L., Ferro, J., & Dunlap, G. (1994). Preferred curricular activities and reduced problem behaviors in students with intellectual disabilities. *Journal of Applied Behavior Analysis, 27*, 493–504.

Foxx, R. M., & Bittle, R. G. (1989). *Thinking it through: Teaching a problem-solving strategy for community living*. Champaign, IL: Research Press.

Foxx, R. M., & Faw, G. D. (2000). The pursuit of actual problem-solving behavior: An opportunity for behavior analysis. *Behavior and Social Issues, 10*, 71–81.

Foxx, R. M., Faw, G. D., Taylor, S., Davis, P. K., & Fulia, R. (1993). "Would I be able to . . . "? Teaching clients to assess the availability of their community living style preferences. *American Journal of Mental Retardation, 98*, 235–248.

Frankland, H. C., Turnbull, A. P., Wehmeyer, M. L., & Blackmountain, L. (2004). An exploration of the self-determination construct and disability as it relates to the Diné (Navajo) culture. *Education and Training in Developmental Disabilities, 39*, 191–205.

Fredericksen, L. W., & Fredericksen, C. B. (1975). Teacher-determined and self-determined token reinforcement in a special education classroom. *Behavior Therapy, 6*, 310–314.

Fujiki, M., & Brinton, B. (1993). Growing old with mental retardation: The language of survivors. *Topics in Language Disorders, 13*(3), 77–89.

Gardner, D. C., & Gardner, P. L. (1978). Goal setting and learning in the high school resource room. *Adolescence, 13*, 489–493.

Gettinger, M. (1985). Effects of teacher-directed versus student-directed instruction and cues versus no cues for improving spelling performance. *Journal of Applied Behavior Analysis, 18*, 167–171.

Gilberts, G. H., Agran, M., Hughes, C., & Wehmeyer, M. (2001). The effects of peer-delivered self-monitoring strategies on the participation of students with severe disabilities in general education classrooms. *Journal of the Association for Persons with Severe Handicaps, 26*, 25–36.

Gothelf, C. R., Crimmins, D. B., Mercer, C. A., & Finocchiaro, P. A. (1994). Teaching choice-making skills to students with dual-sensory impairments. *Teaching Exceptional Children, 26*, 13–15.

Grack, A. (2005). *What states either have, or plan to adopt, legislative or regulatory language requiring secondary transition*. Minneapolis: North Central Regional Resource Center.

Graff, R. B., Gibson, L., & Galiatsatos, G. T. (2006). The impact of high- and low-preference stimuli on vocational and academic performances of youths with severe disabilities. *Journal of Applied Behavior Analysis, 39*, 131–135.

Graham, S., & Harris, K. R. (1997). Self-regulation and writing: Where do we go from here? *Contemporary Educational Psychology, 22*, 102–114.

Graham, S., & Harris, K. (2005). *Writing better: Effective strategies for teaching students with learning difficulties.* Baltimore: Brookes.

Graham, S., MacArthur, C., & Schwartz, S. (1995). The effects of goal setting and procedural facilitation on the revising behavior and writing performance of students with writing and learning problems. *Journal of Educational Psychology, 87*, 230–240.

Graham, S., MacArthur, C., Schwartz, S., & Page-Voth, V. (1992). Improving the compositions of students with learning disabilities using a strategy involving product and process goal setting. *Exceptional Children, 58*, 322–334.

Green, C. W., Gardner, S. M., & Reid, D. H. (1997). Increasing indices of happiness among people with profound multiple disabilities: A program replication and component analysis. *Journal of Applied Behavior Analysis, 30*, 217–228.

Green, C. W., Middleton, S. G., & Reid, D. H. (2000). Embedded evaluation of preferences sampled from person-centered plans for people with profound multiple disabilities. *Journal of Applied Behavior Analysis, 33*, 639–642.

Greene, G., & Kochhar-Bryant, C. A. (2003). *Pathways to successful transition for youth with disabilities.* Upper Saddle River, NJ: Pearson Merrill Prentice Hall.

Grossi, T. A., & Heward, W. L. (1998). Using self-evaluation to improve the work productivity of trainees in a community-based restaurant training program. *Education and Training in Mental Retardation and Developmental Disabilities, 33*, 248–263.

Guerra, N. G., Moore, A., & Slaby, R. G. (1995). *Viewpoints: A guide to conflict resolution and decision making for adolescents.* Champaign, IL: Research Press.

Gumpel, T. P., Tappe, P., & Araki, C. (2000). Comparison of social problem-solving abilities among adults with and without developmental disabilities. *Education and Training in Mental Retardation and Developmental Disabilities, 35*, 259–268.

Guralnick, M. J. (1976). Solving complex perceptual discrimination problems: Techniques for the development of problem solving strategies. *American Journal of Mental Deficiency, 18*, 18–25.

Hagner, D., & Salomone, P. R. (1989). Issues in career decision making for workers with developmental disabilities. *The Career Development Quarterly, 38*, 148–159.

Hagopian, L. P., Long, E. S., & Rush, K. S. (2004). Preference assessment procedures for individuals with developmental disabilities. *Behavior Modification, 28*, 668–677.

Halpern, A. S. (1994). The transition of youth with disabilities to adult life: A position statement of the Division on Career Development and Transition, The Council for Exceptional Children. *Career Development for Exceptional Individuals, 17*, 115–124.

Halpern, A. S., Herr, C. M., Wolf, N. K., Doren, B., Johnson, M. D., & Lawson, J. D. (1997). *Next S.T.E.P.: Student transition and educational planning.* Austin, TX: Pro-Ed.

Hanel, F., & Martin, G. (1980). Self-monitoring, self-administration of token reinforcement, and goal setting to improve work rates with retarded clients. *International Journal of Rehabilitation Research, 3*, 505–517.

Hanley, G. P., Iwata, B. A., & Roscoe, E. M. (2006). Some determinants of changes in preference over time. *Journal of Applied Behavior Analysis, 39*, 189–202.

Harchik, A. E., Sherman, J. A., Sheldon, J. B., & Bannerman, D. J. (1993). Choice and control: New opportunities for people with developmental disabilities. *Annals of Clinical Psychiatry, 5*, 151–161.

Haring, T. G., Breen, C. G., Weiner, J., Kennedy, C. H., & Bednersh, F. (1995). Using video-tape modeling to facilitate generalized purchasing skills. *Journal of Behavioral Education, 5*, 29–53.

Haring, T. G., Kennedy, C. H., Adams, M. J., & Pitts-Conway, V. (1987). Teaching generalization of purchasing skills across community settings to autistic youth using videotape modeling. *Journal of Applied Behavior Analysis, 20*, 89–96.

Harry, B., Rueda, R., & Kalyanpur, M. (1999). Cultural reciprocity in sociocultural perspective: Adapting the normalization principle for family collaboration. *Exceptional Children, 66*, 123–136.

Hayden, M. F., & Nelis, T. (2002). Self-advocacy. In R. L. Schalock, P. C. Baker, & M. D. Crosser (Eds.), *Embarking on a new century: Mental retardation at the end of the 20th century* (pp. 221–233). Washington, DC: American Association on Mental Retardation.

Healey, K., & Masterpasqua, F. (1992). Interpersonal cognitive problem solving among children with mild mental retardation. *American Journal of Mental Retardation, 96*, 367–372.

Helland, C. D., Paluck, R. J., & Klein, M. (1976). A comparison of self- and external reinforcement with the trainable mentally retarded. *Mental Retardation, 14*, 22–23.

Hickson, L., Golden, H., Khemka, I., Urv, T., & Yamusah, S. (1998). A closer look at interpersonal decision making in adults with and without mental retardation. *American Journal of Mental Retardation, 103*, 209–224.

Hickson, L., & Khemka, I. (1999). Decision making and mental retardation. In L. Glidden (Ed.), *International review of research in mental retardation* (Vol. 22, pp. 227–265). San Diego, CA: Academic Press.

Holburn, S. (2002). How science can evaluate and enhance person-centered planning. *Research and Practice for Persons with Severe Disabilities, 27*, 250–260.

Holburn, S., Jacobson, J. W., Schwartz, A. W., Flory, M. J., & Vietze, P. M. (2004). The Willowbrook futures project: A longitudinal analysis of person-centered planning. *American Journal of Mental Retardation, 109*, 63–76.

Hughes, C. (1992). Teaching self-instruction utilizing multiple exemplars to produce generalized problem solving by individuals with severe mental retardation. *American Journal of Mental Retardation, 97*, 302–314.

Hughes, C. (1997). Self-instruction. In M. Agran (Ed.), *Student-directed learning: Teaching self-determination skills* (pp. 144–170). Pacific Grove, CA: Brooks/Cole.

Hughes, C., & Carter, E. W. (2000). *The transition handbook: Strategies high school teachers use that work!* Baltimore: Brookes.

Hughes, C., Copeland, S. R., Agran, M., Wehmeyer, M. L., Rodi, M. S., & Presley, J. A. (2002). Using self-monitoring to improve performance in general education high school classes. *Education and Training in Mental Retardation and Developmental Disabilities, 37*, 262–272.

Hughes, C., Harmer, M. L., Killian, D. J., & Niarhos, F. (1995). The effects of multiple-exemplar self-instructional training on high school students' generalized conversational interactions. *Journal of Applied Behavior Analysis, 28*, 201–218.

Hughes, C., Hugo, K., & Blatt, J. (1996). A self-instructional intervention for teaching generalized problem solving within a functional task sequence. *American Journal of Mental Retardation, 100*, 565–579.

Hughes, C., & Lloyd, J. W. (1993). An analysis of self-management. *Journal of Behavioral Education, 3*, 405–425.

Hughes, C., & Petersen, D. (1989). Utilizing a self-instructional training package to increase on-task behavior and work performance. *Education and Training in Mental Retardation, 24,* 114–120.

Hughes, C., Pitkin, S. E., & Lorden, S. W. (1998). Assessing preferences and choices of persons with severe and profound mental retardation. *Education and Training in Mental Retardation and Developmental Disabilities, 33,* 299–316.

Hughes, C., Rung, L. L., Wehmeyer, M. L., Agran, M., Copeland, S. R., & Hwang, B. (2000). Self-prompted communication book use to increase social interaction among high school students. *Journal of the Association for Persons with Severe Disabilities, 25,* 153–166.

Hughes, C., & Rusch, F. R. (1989). Teaching supported employees with severe mental retardation to solve problems. *Journal of Applied Behavior Analysis, 22,* 365–372.

Hunt, P., Alwell, M., & Goetz, L. (1991). Establishing conversational exchanges with family and friends: Moving from training to meaningful communication. *Journal of Special Education, 25,* 305–319.

Hutchins, M. P., & Renzaglia, A. M. (1990). Developing a longitudinal vocational training program. In F. R. Rusch (Ed.), *Supported employment: Models, methods, and issues* (pp. 365–380). Champaign, IL: Sycamore Press.

Individuals with Disabilities Education Act (IDEA) of 1990, PL 101-476, 20 U.S.C. §§ 1400 *et seq.*

Irvine, B. A., Erickson, A. M., Singer, G., & Stahlberg, D. (1992). A coordinated program to transfer self-management skills from school to home. *Education and Training in Mental Retardation, 27*(3), 241–254.

Jitendra, A. K., Hoppes, M. K., & Zin, Y. P. (2000). Enhancing main idea comprehension for students with learning problems: The role of summarization strategy and self-monitoring instruction. *Journal of Special Education, 34,* 127–139.

Johnson, D. R. (2005). Key provisions on transition: A comparison of IDEA 1997 and IDEA 2004. *Career Development for Exceptional Individuals, 28,* 60–63.

Johnson, L. A., & Graham, S. (1990). Goal setting and its application with exceptional learners. *Preventing School Failure, 34,* 4–8.

Johnson, L., Graham, S., & Harris, K. R. (1997). The effects of goal setting and self-instruction on learning a reading comprehension strategy: A study with students with learning disabilities. *Journal of Learning Disabilities, 30,* 80–91.

Johnston, M. B., Whitman, T. L., & Johnson, M. (1980). Teaching addition and subtraction to mentally retarded children: A self-instruction program. *Applied Research in Mental Retardation, 1,* 141–160.

Joyce, B., & Weil, M. (1980). *Models of teaching* (2nd ed.). Englewood Cliffs, NJ: Prentice Hall.

Kalyanpur, M., & Harry, B. (2004). Impact of the social construction of LD on culturally diverse families: A response to Reid and Valle. *Journal of Learning Disabilities, 37,* 530–533.

Kame'enui, E. J., & Simmons, D. C. (1999). *Toward successful inclusion of students with disabilities: The architecture of instruction.* Arlington, VA: Council for Exceptional Children.

Karvonen, M., Test, D. W., Wood, W. M., Browder, D., & Algozzine, B. (2004). Putting self-determination into practice. *Exceptional Children, 71*(1), 23–41.

Katz, L., Johnson, K. P., & Dalby, J. T. (1981). Teaching nutrition to the developmentally handicapped using computer assisted instruction. *British Journal of Mental Subnormality, 27,* 23–25.

Kaufman, K. F., & O'Leary, K. D. (1972). Reward, cost, and self-evaluation procedures for disruptive adolescents in a psychiatric hospital school. *Journal of Applied Behavior Analysis, 5,* 292–309.

Kennedy, C. H., & Haring, T. (1993). Teaching choice making during social interactions to students with profound multiple disabilities. *Journal of Applied Behavior Analysis, 26*, 63–76.

Keogh, D. A., Faw, G. D., Whitman, T. L., & Reid, D. (1984). Enhancing leisure skills in severely retarded adolescents through a self-instructional treatment package. *Analysis and Intervention in Developmental Disabilities, 4*, 333–351.

Keogh, D. A., Whitman, T. L., & Maxwell, S. E. (1988). Self-instruction versus external instruction: Individual differences and training effectiveness. *Cognitive Therapy and Research, 12*, 591–610.

Kern, L., Dunlap, G., Childs, K. E., & Clarke, S. (1994). Use of a classwide self-monitoring program to improve the behavior of students with emotional and behavioral disorders. *Education and Treatment of Children, 17*(3), 445–458.

Kern, L., Mantegna, M. E., Vorndan, C. M., Bailin, D., & Hilt, A. (2001). Choice of task sequence to reduce problem behaviors. *Journal of Positive Behavior Interventions, 3*, 3–10.

Khemka, I. (2000). Increasing independent decision-making skills of women with mental retardation in simulated interpersonal situations of abuse. *American Journal of Mental Retardation, 105*, 387–401.

Khemka, I., & Hickson, L. (2000). Decision making by adults with mental retardation in simulated situations of abuse. *Mental Retardation, 38*, 15–26.

Khemka, I., Hickson, L., & Reynolds, G. (2005). Evaluation of a decision-making curriculum designed to empower women with mental retardation to resist abuse. *American Journal of Mental Retardation, 110*, 193–204.

Kirkland, K., & Caughlin-Carver, J. (1982). Maintenance and generalization of assertive skills. *Education and Training in Mental Retardation, 17*, 313–318.

Kish, M. (1991). Counseling adolescents with LD. *Intervention in School and Clinic, 27*, 20–24.

Kling, B. (2000). ASSERT yourself: Helping students of all ages develop self-advocacy skills. *Teaching Exceptional Children, 32*, 66–70.

Koegel, R. L., Dyer, K., & Bell, L. K. (1987). The influence of child-preferred activities on autistic children's social behavior. *Journal of Applied Behavior Analysis, 20*, 243–252.

Kohn, A. (1993). Choices for children: Why and how to let students decide. *Phi Delta Kappan, 75*, 8–20.

Koorland, M. A., & Cooke, J. E. (1990). Using fast-food restaurants for consumer education. *Teaching Exceptional Children, 22*, 28–29.

Korinek, L., & Polloway, E. A. (1993). Social skills: Review and implications for instruction for students with mild mental retardation. In R. A. Gable & S. F. Warren (Eds.), *Strategies for teaching students with mild to severe mental retardation* (pp. 71–97). Baltimore: Brookes.

LaFromboise, T., Coleman, H. L., & Gerton, J. (1993). Psychological impact of biculturalism: Evidence and theory. *Psychological Bulletin, 114*, 395–412.

Lancioni, G. E., Oliva, D., Pellegrino, A., & Soresi, S. (1998). A person with intellectual and visual disabilities achieving independent task performance through a self-operated instruction system. *International Journal of Rehabilitation Research, 21*, 231–235.

Lancioni, G. E., O'Reilly, M. F., & Emerson, E. (1996). A review of choice research with people with severe and profound developmental disabilities. *Research in Developmental Disabilities, 17*, 391–411.

Lancioni, G. E., O'Reilly, M. F., & Oliva, D. (2002). Engagement in cooperative and individual tasks: Assessing the performance and preferences of persons with multiple disabilities. *Journal of Visual Impairment and Blindness, 96*, 50–53.

Lancioni, G. E., O'Reilly, M. F., Oliva, D., & Coppa, M. M. (2001). A microswitch for vocalization responses to foster environmental control in children with multiple disabilities. *Journal of Intellectual Disability Research, 45,* 271–275.

Lancioni, G. E., van den Hof, E., Boelens, H., Rocha, N., & Seedhouse, P. (1998). A computer-based system providing pictorial instructions and prompts to promote task performance in persons with severe developmental disabilities. *Behavioral Interventions, 13,* 111–122.

Langone, J., Shade, J., Clees, T. J., & Day, T. (1999). Effects of multimedia instruction on teaching functional discrimination skills to students with moderate/severe intellectual disabilities. *International Journal of Disability, Development and Education, 46,* 493–513.

Lattimore, L. P., Parsons, M. B., & Reid, D. H. (2003). Assessing preferred work among adults with autism beginning supported jobs: Identification of constant and alternating task preferences. *Behavioral Interventions, 18,* 161–177.

Leake, D., & Black, R. (2005). Cultural and linguistic diversity: Implications for transition personnel. *National Center on Secondary Education and Transition, Essential Tools: October 2005.* Retrieved January 12, 2006, from *www.ncset.org/publications/essentialtools/diversity/default.asp*

Leake, D., Black, R., & Roberts, K. (2004). Assumptions in transition planning: Are they culturally sensitive? *Impact, 16*(3), 28–30.

Lee, S. H., & Wehmeyer, M. L. (2004). A review of the Korean literature related to self-determination: Future directions and practices for promoting the self-determination of students with disabilities. *Korean Journal of Special Education, 38,* 369–390.

Lehman, J. P., Davies, T. G., & Laurin, K. M. (2000). Listening to student voices about postsecondary education. *Teaching Exceptional Children, 32,* 60–65.

Lehmann, J. P., Bassett, D. S., & Sands, D. J. (1999). Students' participation in transition-related actions: A qualitative study. *Remedial and Special Education, 20,* 160–169.

Lenz, B. K., Ehren, B. J., & Smiley, L. R. (1991). A goal attainment approach to improve completion of project-type assignments by learning-disabled adolescents. *Learning Disabilities Research and Practice, 6,* 166–176.

Levendoski, L. S., & Cartledge, G. (2000). Self-monitoring for elementary school children with serious emotional disturbances: Classroom applications for increased academic responding. *Behavioral Disorders, 25,* 211–224.

Lloyd, J. W., Hallahan, D. P., Kosiewicz, M. M., & Kneedler, R. D. (1982). Reactive effects of self-assessment and self-recording on attention to task and academic productivity. *Learning Disabilities Quarterly, 5,* 216–227.

Locke, E. A., & Latham, G. P. (1990). *A theory of goal setting and task performance.* Englewood, NJ: Prentice Hall.

Locke, E. A., & Latham, G. P. (2002). Building a practically useful theory of goal setting and task motivation: A 35-year odyssey. *American Psychologist, 57,* 705–717.

Logan, K. R., & Gast, D. L. (2001). Conducting preference assessments and reinforcer testing for individuals with profound multiple disabilities: Issues and procedures. *Exceptionality, 9,* 123–134.

Lohrmann-O'Rourke, S., & Browder, D. M. (1998). Empirically based methods to assess the preferences of individuals with severe disabilities. *American Journal of Mental Retardation, 103,* 146–161.

Lohrmann-O'Rourke, S., Browder, D. M., & Brown, F. (2000). Guidelines for conducting socially valid systematic preference assessments. *Journal of the Association for Persons with Severe Handicaps, 25,* 42–53.

Lohrmann-O'Rourke, S., & Gomez, O. (2001). Integrating preference assessment within the transition process to create meaningful school-to-life outcomes. *Exceptionality, 9,* 157–174.

Lovitt, T. C., & Curtiss, K. A. (1969). Academic response rate as a function of teacher and self-imposed contingencies. *Journal of Applied Behavior Analysis, 2,* 49–53.

Lovitt, T. C., Cushing, S. S., & Stump, C. S. (1994). High school students rate their IEPs: Low opinion and lack of ownership. *Intervention in School and Clinic, 30,* 34–38.

Luria, A. R. (1961). Psychological studies of mental deficiency in the Soviet Union. In N. R. Ellis (Ed.), *Handbook of mental deficiency* (pp. 243–275). New York: McGraw-Hill.

Mahoney, M. J., Moura, N. G. M., & Wade, T. C. (1973). The relative efficacy of self-reward, self-punishment, and self-monitoring techniques for weight loss. *Journal of Consulting and Clinical Psychology, 40,* 404–407.

Malott, R. W. (1984). Rule-governed behavior, self-management, and the developmentally disabled: A theoretical analysis. *Analysis and Intervention in Developmental Disabilities, 4,* 199–209.

Margalit, M. (1991). Promoting classroom adjustment and social skills for students with mental retardation within an experimental and control group design. *Exceptionality, 2,* 195–204.

Margalit, M. (1995). Effects of social skills training for students with an intellectual disability. *International Journal of Disability, Development and Education, 42,* 75–85.

Marshall, L. H., Martin, J. E., Maxson, L., & Jerman, P. (1997). *Choosing employment goals.* Longmont, CO: Sopris West.

Martin, G. L., & Hrydowy, E. R. (1989). Self-monitoring and self-managed reinforcement procedures for improving work productivity of developmentally disabled workers. *Behavior Modification, 13,* 323–339.

Martin, J. E., Elias-Burger, S., & Mithaug, D. E. (1987). Acquisition and maintenance of time-based task change sequence. *Education and Training in Mental Retardation, 22,* 250–255.

Martin, J. E., Greene, B. A., & Borland, B. J. (2004). Secondary students' involvement in their IEP meetings: Administrators' perceptions. *Career Development for Exceptional Individuals, 27,* 177–188.

Martin, J. E., & Marshall, L. H. (1995). ChoiceMaker: A comprehensive self-determination transition program. *Intervention in School and Clinic, 30*(3), 147–156.

Martin, J. E., Marshall, L. H., & Maxson, L. L. (1993). Transition policy: Infusing self determination and self-advocacy into transition programs. *Career Development for Exceptional Individuals, 16,* 53–61.

Martin, J. E., Marshall, L. H., Maxson, L. M., & Jerman, P. L. (1997). *The Self-Directed IEP.* Longmont, CO: Sopris West.

Martin, J. E., Marshall, L. H., & Sale, P. (2004). A 3-year study of middle, junior high, and high school IEP meetings. *Exceptional Children, 70,* 285–297.

Martin, J. E., Marshall, L. H., Wray, D., Obrien, J., Wells, L., Olvey, G. H., et al. (2004). *Choose and take action: Finding the right job for you.* Longmont, CO: Sopris West Educational Services.

Martin, J. E., Mithaug, D. E., Cox, P., Peterson, L. Y., Van Dycke, J. L., & Cash, M. E. (2003). Increasing self-determination: Teaching students to plan, work, evaluate, and adjust. *Exceptional Children, 69*(4), 431–447.

Martin, J. E., Mithaug, D. E., & Frazier, E. S. (1992). Effects of picture referencing on PVC chair, love seat, and settee assemblies by students with mental retardation. *Research in Developmental Disabilities, 13,* 267–286.

Martin, J. E., Mithaug, D. E., Husch, J. V., Frazier, E. S., & Marshall, L. H. (2003). The effects of optimal opportunities and adjustments on job choices of adults with severe disabilities. In D. E. Mithaug, D. K. Mithaug, M. Agran, J. E. Martin, & M. L. Wehmeyer (Eds.), *Self-determined learning theory: Construction, verification, and evaluation* (pp. 188–205). Mahwah, NJ: Erlbaum.

Martin, J. E., Mithaug, D. E., Oliphant, J. H., Husch, J. V., & Frazier, E. S. (2002). *Self-directed employment: A handbook for transition teachers and employment specialists*. Baltimore: Brookes.

Martin, J. E., Rusch, F. R., James, V. L., Decker, P. J., & Trtol, K. A. (1982). The use of picture cues to establish self-control in the preparation of complex meals by mentally retarded adults. *Applied Research in Mental Retardation, 3*, 105–119.

Martin, J. E., Valenzuela, R., Woods, L., & Borland, B. (2004). Self-directed transition and employment. In J. L. Matson, R. B. Laud, & M. L. Matson (Eds.), *Behavior modification for persons with developmental disabilities* (Vol. 2, pp. 133–171). Kingston, NY: National Association for the Dually Diagnosed.

Martin, J. E., Van Dycke, J. L., Christensen, W. R., Greene, B. A., Gardner, J. E., & Lovett, D. L. (2006) Increasing student participation in IEP meetings: Establishing the Self-Directed IEP as an evidence-based practice. *Exceptional Children, 72*, 299–316.

Martin, J. E., Van Dycke, J. L., Greene, B. A., Gardner, J. E., Christensen, W. R., Woods, L. L., et al. (2006). Direct observation of teacher-directed IEP meetings: Establishing the need for student IEP meeting instruction. *Exceptional Children, 72*, 187–200.

Martin, J. E., Woods, L. L., Sylvester, L., & Gardner, J. E. (2005). A challenge to self-determination: Disagreement between the vocational choices made by individuals with severe disabilities and their caregivers. *Research and Practice for Persons with Severe Disabilities, 30*, 147–153.

Mason, C. Y., Field, S., & Sawilowsky, S. (2004). Implementation of self-determination activities and student participation in IEPs. *Exceptional Children, 70*(4), 441–451.

Mason, C., McGahee-Kovac, M., Johnson, L., & Stillerman, S. (2002). Implementing student-led IEPs: Student participation and student and teacher reactions. *Career Development for Exceptional Individuals, 25*, 171–192.

Masters, J. C. (1968). Effects of social comparison upon subsequent self-reinforcement behavior in children. *Journal of Personality and Social Psychology, 10*, 391–401.

Masters, J. C., & Christy, M. D. (1974). Achievement standards for contingent self-reinforcement: Effects of task length and task difficulty. *Child Development, 45*, 9–13.

Masters, J. C., Furman, W., & Barden, R. C. (1977). Effects of achievement standards, tangible rewards, and self-dispensed achievement evaluations on children's task mastery. *Child Development, 48*, 217–224.

Mattie, H. D. (2001). Generalization effects of cognitive strategies conversation training for adults with moderate to severe disabilities. *Education and Training in Mental Retardation and Developmental Disabilities, 36*, 178–187.

McGahee, M., Mason, C., Wallace, T., & Jones, B. (2001). *Student-led IEPs: A guide for student involvement*. Arlington, VA: Council for Exceptional Children.

McGlashing-Johnson, J., Agran, M., Sitlington, P., Cavin, M., & Wehmeyer, M. L. (2003). Enhancing the job performance of youth with moderate to severe cognitive disabilities using the self-determined learning model of instruction. *Research and Practice for Persons with Severe Disabilities, 28*, 194–204.

Mechling, L. C., & Gast, D. L. (1997). Combination audio/visual self-prompting system for teaching chained tasks to students with intellectual disabilities. *Education and Training in Mental Retardation and Developmental Disabilities, 32*, 138–153.

Mechling, L. C., Gast, D. L., & Langone, J. (2002). Computer-based video instruction to teach persons with moderate intellectual disabilities to read grocery aisle signs and locate items. *Journal of Special Education, 35*, 224–240.

Miller, D. L., & Kelly, M. L. (1994). The use of goal setting and contingency contracting for improving children's homework performance. *Journal of Applied Behavior Analysis, 27*, 73–84.

Miner, C. A., & Bates, P. E. (1997). The effect of person-centered planning activities on the IEP/transition-planning process. *Education and Training in Mental Retardation and Developmental Disabilities, 32*, 105–112.

Mithaug, D. E. (1991). *Self-determined kids: Raising satisfied and successful children.* Lexington, MA: Lexington Books.

Mithaug, D. E. (1993). *Self-regulation theory: How optimal adjustment maximizes gain.* Westport, CT: Praeger.

Mithaug, D. E. (1996a). *Equal opportunity theory.* Thousand Oaks, CA: Sage.

Mithaug, D. E. (1996b). The optimal prospects principle: A theoretical basis for rethinking instructional practices for self-determination. In D. J. Sands & M. L. Wehmeyer (Eds.), *Self-determination across the life span: Independence and choice for people with disabilities* (pp. 147–165). Baltimore: Brookes.

Mithaug, D. E. (1998). Your right, my obligation? *Journal of the Association for Persons with Severe Disabilities, 23*, 41–43.

Mithaug, D. E. (2005). On persistent pursuits of self-interests. *Research and Practice for Persons with Severe Disabilities, 30*, 163–167.

Mithaug, D. E., Campeau, P., & Wolman, J. (1992). *Self-determination assessment project.* Unpublished grant proposal.

Mithaug, D. E., & Hanawalt, D. A. (1978). The validation of procedures to assess prevocational task preferences in three severely retarded young adults. *Journal of Applied Behavior Analysis, 11*, 153–162.

Mithaug, D. E., & Mar, D. K. (1980). The relation between choosing and working prevocational tasks in two severely retarded young adults. *Journal of Applied Behavior Analysis, 13*, 177–182.

Mithaug, D. E., Martin, J. E., & Agran, M. (1987). Adaptability instruction: The goal of transitional programming. *Exceptional Children, 53*, 500–505.

Mithaug, D. E., Martin, J. E., Agran, M., Husch J. V., & Rusch, F. R. (1988). *When will persons in supported employment need less support?* Colorado Springs, CO: Ascent Publications.

Mithaug, D. E., Martin, J. E., Agran, M., & Rusch, F. R. (1988). *Why special education graduates fail: How to teach them to succeed.* Colorado Springs: CO: Ascent.

Mithaug, D. E., Mithaug, D. K., Agran, M., Martin, J. E., & Wehmeyer, M. L. (Eds.). (2003). *Self-determined learning theory: Construction, verification, and evaluation.* Mahwah, NJ: Erlbaum.

Mithaug, D. E., Wehmeyer, M. L., Agran, M., Martin, J., & Palmer, S. (1998). The self-determined learning model of instruction: Engaging students to solve their learning problems. In M. L. Wehmeyer & D. J. Sands (Eds.), *Making it happen: Student involvement in educational planning, decision making and instruction* (pp. 299–328). Baltimore: Brookes.

Mithaug, D. K., & Mithaug, D. E. (2003). The effects of teacher-directed versus student-directed instruction on the self-management of young children with disabilities. *Journal of Applied Behavior Analysis, 36*, 133–136.

Moore, S. C., Agran, M., & Fodor-Davis, J. (1989). Using self-management strategies to increase the production rates of workers with severe handicaps. *Education and Training in Mental Retardation, 24*, 324–332.

Morgan, P. L. (2006). Increasing task engagement using preference or choice-making: Some behavioral and methodological factors affecting their efficacy as classroom interventions. *Remedial and Special Education, 27*, 176–187.

Morningstar, M. E., Turnbull, A. P., & Turnbull, H. R. (1995). What do students with disabilities tell us about the importance of family involvement in the transition from school to adult life? *Exceptional Children, 62*, 249–260.

Nelson, J. R., Smith, D. J., & Colvin, G. (1995). The effects of peer-mediated self-evaluation procedures on playground behavior. *Journal of Remedial and Special Education, 16*, 117–125.

Nelson, W. J., Jr., & Birkimer, J. C. (1978). The role of self-instruction and self-reinforcement in the modification of impulsivity. *Journal of Consulting and Clinical Psychology, 46*, 183.

Neubert, D. A., Danehey, A. J., & Taymans, J. M. (1990). Vocational interests, job tryouts and employment outcomes of individuals with mild disabilities in a time-limited transition program. *Vocational Evaluation and Work Adjustment Bulletin, 23*, 17–23.

Newman, B., Buffington, D. M., & Hemmers, N. S. (1996). External and self-reinforcement used to increase the appropriate conversation of autistic teenagers. *Education and Training in Mental Retardation and Developmental Disabilities, 31*, 304–309.

Newton, M., & Duda, J. (1993). Elite adolescent athletes' achievement goals and beliefs concerning success in tennis. *Journal of Sport and Exercise Psychology, 15*, 437–459.

Nietupski, J., Hamre-Nietupski, S., Green, K., Varnum-Teeter, K., Twedt, B., LePera, D., et al. (1986). Self-initiated and sustained leisure activity participation by students with moderate/severe handicaps. *Education and Training of the Mentally Retarded, 21*, 259–264.

Nirje, B. (1972). The right to self-determination. In W. Wolfensberger (Ed.), *Normalization: The principle of normalization* (pp. 176–193). Toronto: National Institute on Mental Retardation.

O'Brien, C. L., & O'Brien, J. (2002). The origins of person-centered planning: A community of practice perspective. In S. Holburn & P. M. Vietze (Eds.), *Person-centered planning* (pp. 3–27). Baltimore: Brookes.

O'Brien, C. L., O'Brien, J., & Mount, B. (1997). Person-centered planning has arrived. Or has it? *Mental Retardation, 35*, 480–484.

O'Brien, J. (2002). Person-centered planning as a contributing factor in organizational and social change. *Research and Practice for Persons with Severe Disabilities, 27*, 261–264.

Ohtake, Y., & Wehmeyer, M. L. (2004). Applying the self-determination theory to Japanese special education contexts: A four-step model. *Journal of Policy and Practice in Intellectual Disabilities, 1*, 169–178.

O'Reilly, M. F., Lancioni, G. E., Gardiner, M., Tiernan, R., & Lacy, C. (2002). Using a problem-solving approach to teach classroom skills to a student with moderate intellectual disabilities within regular classroom settings. *International Journal of Disability, Development and Education, 49*, 95–104.

O'Reilly, M. F., Lancioni, G. E., & Kierans, I. (2000). Teaching leisure social skills to adults with moderate mental retardation: An analysis of acquisition, generalization, and maintenance. *Education and Training in Mental Retardation and Developmental Disabilities, 35*, 250–258.

O'Reilly, M. F., Lancioni, G. E., & O'Kane, N. (2000). Using a problem-solving approach to teach social skills to workers with brain injuries in supported employment settings. *Journal of Vocational Rehabilitation, 14*, 187–194.

O'Reilly, M., Tiernan, R., Lancioni, G., Lacey, C., Hillery, J., & Gardiner, M. (2002). Use of self-monitoring and delayed feedback to increase on-task behavior in a post-institutionalized child within regular classroom settings. *Education and Treatment of Children, 25*, 91–102.

Orkwis, R., & McLane, K. (1998). A curriculum every student can use: Design principles for student access. *ERIC/OSEP Topical Brief*. Reston, VA: Council for Exceptional Children.

Pace, G., Ivancic, M., Edwards, G., Iwata, B., & Page, T. (1985). Assessment of stimulus preference and reinforcer value with profoundly retarded individuals. *Journal of Applied Behavior Analysis, 18*, 249–255.

Page-Voth, V., & Graham, S. (1999). Effects of goal setting and strategy use on the writing performance and self-efficacy of students with writing and learning problems. *Journal of Educational Psychology, 91*, 230–240.

Palmer, S., & Wehmeyer, M. L. (2003). Promoting self-determination in early elementary school: Teaching self-regulated problem-solving and goal setting skills. *Remedial and Special Education, 24*, 115–126.

Palmer, S. B., Wehmeyer, M. L., Gipson, K., & Agran, M. (2004). Promoting access to the general curriculum by teaching self-determination skills. *Exceptional Children, 70*, 427–439.

Park, H. S., & Gaylord-Ross, R. (1989). A problem-solving approach to social skills training in employment settings with mentally retarded youth. *Journal of Applied Behavior Analysis, 22*, 373–380.

Parsons, M., McCarn, J., & Reid, D. (1993). Evaluating and increasing meal-related choice throughout a service setting for people with severe disabilities. *Journal of the Association for Persons with Severe Handicaps, 18*, 253–260.

Parsons, M., & Reid, D. (1990). Assessing food preferences among persons with profound mental retardation: Providing opportunities to make choices. *Journal of Applied Behavior Analysis, 23*, 183–195.

Parsons, M. B., Reid, D. H., & Green, C. W. (2001). Situational assessment of task preferences among adults with multiple severe disabilities in supported work. *Journal of the Association for Persons with Severe Handicaps, 26*, 50–55.

Parsons, R., Reid, D., Reynolds, J., & Bumgarner, M. (1990). Effects of chosen versus assigned jobs on the work performance of persons with severe handicaps. *Journal of Applied Behavior Analysis, 23*, 253–258.

Perske, R. (1972). The dignity of risk. In W. Wolfensberger (Ed.), *Normalization: The principle of normalization in human services* (pp. 194–200). Toronto: National Institute on Mental Retardation.

Peterson, M. (1996). Community learning in inclusive schools. In S. Stainback & W. Stainback (Eds.), *Inclusion: A guide for educators* (pp. 271–293). Baltimore: Brookes.

Pierce, K. L., & Schreibman, L. (1994). Teaching daily living skills to children with autism in unsupervised settings through pictorial self-management. *Journal of Applied Behavior Analysis, 27*, 471–481.

Powers, L. E. (2005). Self-determination by individuals with severe disabilities: Limitations or excuses? *Research and Practice for Persons with Severe Disabilities, 30*, 168–172.

Powers, L. E., Sowers, J. A., Turner, A., Nesbitt, M., Knowles, E., & Ellison, R. (1996). TAKE CHARGE!: A model for promoting self-determination among adolescents with challenges. In L. E. Powers, G. H. S. Singer, & J. Sowers (Eds.), *On the road to autonomy: Pro-*

moting self-competence in children and youth with disabilities (pp. 241–270). Baltimore: Brookes.

Powers, L. E., Turner, A., Matuszewski, J., Wilson, R., & Loesch, C. (1999). A qualitative analysis of student involvement in transition planning. *Journal for Vocational Special Needs Education, 21,* 18–26.

Powers, L. E., Turner, A., Matuszewski, J., Wilson, R., & Phillips, A. (2001). TAKE CHARGE for the future: A controlled field test of a model to promote student involvement in transition planning. *Career Development for Exceptional Individuals, 24,* 89–103.

Powers, L. E., Turner, A., Westwood, D., Loesch, C., Brown, A., & Rowland, C. (1998). TAKE CHARGE for the future: A student-directed approach to transition planning. In M. L. Wehmeyer and D. J. Sands (Eds.), *Making it happen: Student involvement in education planning, decision making, and instruction* (pp. 187–210). Baltimore: Brookes.

President's Commission on Excellence in Special Education. (2003). *A new era: Revitalizing special education for children and their families.* Washington, DC: U.S. Department of Special Education and Rehabilitative Services.

Rachlin, H. (1978). Self-control: Part I. In A. C. Catania & T. A. Brigham (Eds.), *Handbook of applied behavior analysis: Social and instructional processes* (pp. 246–258). New York: Irvington.

Rakos, R. F. (1991). *Assertive behavior: Theory, research and training.* London: Routledge.

Raskind, M. H., Goldberg, R. J., Higgins, E. L., & Herman, K. L. (2002). Teaching life success to students with LD: Lessons learned from a 20-year study. *Intervention in School and Clinic, 37,* 201–208.

Rawlings, M., Dowse, L., & Shaddock, A. (1995). Increasing the involvement of people with intellectual disability in choice making situations: A practical approach. *International Journal of Disability, Development and Education, 42,* 137–153.

Reid, D. H., Parsons, M. B., & Green, C. W. (1991). *Providing choices and preferences for persons who have severe handicaps.* Morganton, NC: Habilitative Management Consultants.

Reinecke, D. R., Newman, B., & Meinberg, D. L. (1999). Self-management of sharing in three pre-schoolers with autism. *Education and Training in Mental Retardation and Developmental Disabilities, 34,* 312–317.

Rhode, G., Morgan, D. P., & Young, K. R. (1983). Generalization and maintenance of treatment gains of behaviorally handicapped students from resource rooms to regular classrooms using self-evaluation procedures. *Journal of Applied Behavior Analysis, 16,* 171–187.

Rich, A. R., & Schroeder, H. E. (1976). Research issues in assertiveness training. *Psychological Bulletin, 83,* 1084–1096.

Riffel, L. A., Wehmeyer, M. L., Turnbull, A. P., Lattimore, J., Davies, D. K., Stock, S., et al. (2005). Promoting independent performance of transition-related tasks using a palmtop PC-based self-directed visual and auditory prompting system. *Journal of Special Education Technology, 20*(2), 5–14.

Rimm, D. C., & Masters, J. C. (1979). *Behavior therapy: Techniques and empirical findings.* New York: Academic Press.

Roffman, A. (1994). Social skills training. In C. A. Michaels (Ed.), *Transition strategies for persons with learning disabilities* (pp. 185–211). San Diego: Singular Publications.

Romaniuk, C., & Miltenberger, R. G. (2001). The influence of preference and choice of activity on problem behavior. *Journal of Positive Behavior Interventions, 3,* 152–159.

Rusch, F. R., Martin, J. E., Lagomarcino, T. R., & White, D. M. (1987). Teaching task sequencing via verbal mediation. *Education and Training in Mental Retardation, 22,* 229–235.

Rusch, F. R., McKee, M., Chadsey-Rusch, J., & Renzaglia, A. (1988). Teaching a student with severe handicaps to self-instruct: A brief report. *Education and Training in Mental Retardation, 23*, 51–58.

Rusch, F. R., Morgan, T. K., Martin, J. E., Riva, M., & Agran, M. (1985). Competitive employment: Teaching mentally retarded employees self-instructional strategies. *Applied Research in Mental Retardation, 6*, 389–407.

Ruth, W. J. (1996). Goal setting and behavior contracting for students with emotional and behavioral difficulties: Analysis of daily, weekly, and total goal attainment. *Psychology in the Schools, 33*, 153–158.

Sainato, D. M., Strain, P. S., Lefebvre, D., & Rapp, N. (1990). The effects of self-evaluation package on the independent work skills of handicapped preschool children. *Exceptional Children, 56*, 540–549.

Salter, A. (1949). *Conditioned reflex therapy*. New York: Farrar, Strauss & Giroux.

Sands, D., & Doll, E. (2005). Teaching goal setting and decision making to students with developmental disabilities. In M. L. Wehmeyer & M. Agran (Eds.), *Mental retardation and intellectual disabilities: Teaching students using innovative and research-based strategies* (pp. 273–296). Washington, DC: American Association on Mental Retardation.

Schaller, J. L., & Szymanski, E. M. (1992). Supported employment, consumer choice, and independence. *Journal of Vocational Rehabilitation, 2*, 45–50.

Schalock, R. L. (1996). Reconsidering the conceptualization and measurement of quality of life. In R. L. Schalock (Ed.), *Quality of life: Vol 1. Conceptualization and measurement* (pp. 123–139). Washington, DC: American Association on Mental Retardation.

Schalock, R. L., Verdugo, M. A., Jenaro, C., Wang, M., Wehmeyer, M., Jiancheng, X., et al. (2005). Cross-cultural study of quality of life indicators. *American Journal of Mental Retardation, 110*(4), 298–311.

Schloss, P. J., Alper, S., & Jayne, D. (1994). Self-determination for persons with disabilities: Choice, risk, and dignity. *Exceptional Children, 60*, 215–225.

Schloss, P. J., & Smith, M. A. (1998). *Applied behavior analysis in the classroom*. Boston: Allyn & Bacon.

Schwartz, A. A., Jacobson, J. W., & Holburn, S. (2000). Defining person centeredness: Results of two consensus methods. *Education and Training in Mental Retardation and Developmental Disabilities, 35*, 235–249.

Schwartzman, L., Martin, G. L., Yu, C. T., & Whiteley, J. (2004). Choice, degree of preference, and happiness indices with persons with intellectual disabilities: A surprising finding. *Education and Training in Developmental Disabilities, 39*, 265–269.

Senatore, V., Matson, J. L., & Kazdin, A. E. (1982). A comparison of behavioral methods to train social skills to mentally retarded adults. *Behavior Therapy, 13*, 313–324.

Senf, G. M. (1976). Future research needs in learning disabilities. In R. P. Anderson & C. G. Halcomb (Eds.), *Learning disabilities/minimal brain dysfunction syndrome* (pp. 249–267). Springfield, IL: Charles C Thomas.

Serna, L. A., & Lau-Smith, J. (1995). Learning with purpose: Self-determination skills for students who are at risk for school and community failure. *Intervention in School and Clinic, 30*(3), 142–146.

Seybert, S., Dunlap, G., & Ferro, J. (1996). The effects of choice making on the problem behaviors of high school students with intellectual disabilities. *Journal of Behavioral Education, 6*, 49–65.

Shapiro, E. S., McGonigle, J. J., & Ollendick, T. H. (1980). An analysis of self-assessment and self-reinforcement in a self-managed token economy with mentally retarded children. *Applied Research in Mental Retardation, 1,* 227–240.

Shevin, M., & Klein, N. K. (1984). The importance of choice making skills for students with severe disabilities. *Journal of the Association for Persons with Severe Handicaps, 9,* 159–166.

Shogren, K. A., Faggella-Luby, M., Bae, S. J., & Wehmeyer, M. L. (2004). The effect of choice-making as an intervention for problem behavior: A meta-analysis. *Journal of Positive Behavior Interventions, 6,* 228–237.

Shore, B. A., Iwata, B. A., Lerman, D. C., & Shirley, M. J. (1994). Assessing and programming generalized behavioral reduction across multiple stimulus parameters. *Journal of Applied Behavior Analysis, 27,* 371–384.

Short, F. J., & Evans, S. W. (1990). Individual differences in cognitive and social problem-solving skills as a function of intelligence. In N. W. Bray (Ed.), *International review of research in mental retardation* (Vol. 16, pp. 89–123). San Diego, CA: Academic Press.

Shure, M. B., Spivack, G., & Jaeger, M. (1972). Problem-solving thinking and adjustment among disadvantaged preschool children. *Child Development, 42,* 1791–1803.

Sigafoos, J., & Dempsey, R. (1992). Assessing choice making among children with multiple disabilities. *Journal of Applied Behavior Analysis, 25,* 747–755.

Sigafoos, J., Roberts, D., Couzens, D., & Kerr, M. (1993). Providing opportunities for choice-making and turn-taking to adults with multiple disabilities. *Journal of Developmental and Physical Disabilities, 5,* 297–310.

Simpson, G., & Weiner, W. (1989). *Oxford English dictionary.* Oxford, UK: Oxford University Press.

Singh, N. N., Lancioni, G. E., O'Reilly, M. F., Molina, E. J., Adkins, A. D., & Oliva, D. (2003). Self-determination during mealtimes through microswitch choice making by an individual with complex multiple disabilities and profound mental retardation. *Journal of Positive Behavior Interventions, 5,* 209–216.

Smith, D. J., & Nelson, J. R. (1997). Goal setting, self-monitoring, and self-evaluation for students with disabilities. In M. Agran (Ed.), *Student-directed learning: Teaching self-determination skills* (pp. 80–110). Pacific Grove, CA: Brooks/Cole.

Smull, M. W. (1998). Revisiting choice. In J. O'Brien & C. L. O'Brien (Eds.), *A little book about person-centered planning* (pp. 37–49). Toronto: Inclusion Press.

Smull, M. W., & Lakin, K. C. (2002). Public policy and person-centered planning. In S. Holburn & P. M. Vietze (Eds.), *Person-centered planning: Research practice and future directions* (pp. 379–397). Baltimore: Brookes.

Snyder, E. P. (2000). *Examining the effects of teaching ninth-grade students receiving special education learning support services to conduct their own IEP meetings.* Unpublished doctoral dissertation, Lehigh University, Bethlehem, PA.

Snyder, E. P. (2002). Teaching students with combined behavioral disorders and mental retardation to lead their own IEP meetings. *Behavioral Disorders, 27,* 340–357.

Snyder, E. P., & Shapiro, E. (1997). Teaching students with emotional disorders the skills to participate in the development of their own IEPs. *Behavioral Disorders, 22,* 246–259.

Sowers, J., & Powers, L. (1995). Enhancing the participation and independence of students with severe physical and multiple disabilities in performing community activities. *Mental Retardation, 33,* 209–220.

Spates, C. R., & Kanfer, F. H. (1977). Self-monitoring, self-evaluation, and self-reinforcement in children's learning: A test of a multistage self-regulation model. *Behavior Therapy, 8,* 9–16.

Spivack, G., & Shure, M. (1974). *Social adjustment of young children*. San Francisco, CA: Jossey-Bass.

Stafford, A. M., Alberto, P. A., Fredrick, L. D., Heflin, L. J., & Heller, K. W. (2002). Preference variability and the instruction of choice making with students with severe intellectual disabilities. *Education and Training in Mental Retardation and Developmental Disabilities, 37*, 70–88.

Stancliffe, R. J. (1997). Community living-unit size, staff presence and residents' choice-making. *Mental Retardation, 35*, 1–9.

Stancliffe, R. J., & Abery, B. H. (1997). Longitudinal study of deinstitutionalization and the exercise of choice. *Mental Retardation, 35*, 159–169.

Stancliffe, R. J., Abery, B. H., & Smith, J. (2000). Personal control and the ecology of community living settings: Beyond living-unit size and type. *American Journal of Mental Retardation, 105*, 431–454.

Stancliffe, R. J., & Wehmeyer, M. L. (1995). Variability in the availability of choice to adults with mental retardation. *Journal of Vocational Rehabilitation, 5*, 319–328.

Stevenson, H. C., & Fantuzzo, J. W. (1984). Application of the "generalization map" to a self-control intervention with school-aged children. *Journal of Applied Behavior Analysis, 17*, 203–212.

Stevenson, H. C., & Fantuzzo, J. W. (1986). The generality of social validity of a competency-based intervention with school-aged children. *Journal of Applied Behavior Analysis, 19*, 269–276.

Stock, S., Davies, D. K., Davies, K. R., & Wehmeyer, M. L. (2006). Evaluation of an application for making palmtop computers accessible to individuals with intellectual disabilities. *Journal of Intellectual and Developmental Disabilities, 31*, 39–46.

Stokes, T., & Baer, D. (1977). An implicit technology of generalization. *Journal of Applied Behavior Analysis, 10*, 349–367.

Storey, K. (2002). Strategies for increasing interactions in supported employment settings: An updated review. *Journal of Vocational Rehabilitation, 17*, 231–237.

Sue, D. W., Bingham, R. P. Porshé-Burke, L., & Vasquez, M. (1999). The diversification of psychology: A multicultural revolution. *American Psychologist, 54*, 1061–1069.

Suto, W. M. I., Clare, I. C. H., Holland, A. J., & Watson, P. C. (2005a). Capacity to make financial decisions among people with mild intellectual disabilities. *Journal of Intellectual Disability Research, 49*, 199–209.

Suto, W. M. I., Clare, I. C. H., Holland, A. J., & Watson, P. C. (2005b). The relationship among three factors affecting the financial decision-making ability of adults with mild intellectual disabilities. *Journal of Intellectual Disability Research, 49*, 210–217.

Sweeney, M. A. (1997). *The effects of self-determination training on student involvement in the IEP process*. Unpublished doctoral dissertation, Florida State University, Tallahassee.

Taber-Doughty, T. (2005). Considering student choice when selecting instructional strategies: A comparison of three prompting systems. *Research in Developmental Disabilities, 26*, 411–432.

Test, D. W., Aspel, N. P., & Everson, J. M. (2006). *Transition methods for youth with disabilities*. Upper Saddle River, NJ: Pearson Merrill Prentice Hall.

Test, D., Fowler, C., Brewer, D., & Wood, W. (2005). A content and methodological review of self-advocacy intervention studies. *Exceptional Children, 72*, 101–125.

Thoma, C. A., Held, M. F., & Sadler, S. (2002). Transition assessment practices in Nevada and Arizona: Are they tied to best practices? *Focus on Autism and Other Developmental Disabilities, 17*, 242–250.

Thomas, J. D. (1976). Accuracy of self-assessment of on-task behavior by elementary school children. *Journal of Applied Behavior Analysis, 9*, 209–210.

Thompson, J. R., Bryant, B. R., Campbell, E. M., Craig, E. M., Hughes, C. M., Rotholz, D. A., et al. (2004). *Supports intensity scale: Users manual.* Washington, DC: American Association on Mental Retardation.

Trainor, A. T. (2002). Self-determination for students with learning disabilities: Is it a universal value? *Qualitative Studies in Education, 15*(6), 711–725.

Trammel, D. L., Schloss, P. T., & Alper, S. (1994). Using self-recording evaluation and graphing to increase completion of homework assignments. *Journal of Learning Disabilities, 27* (2), 75–81.

Trask-Tyler, S. A., Grossi, T. A., & Heward, W. L. (1994). Teaching young adults with developmental disabilities and visual impairments to use tape-recorded recipes: Acquisition, generalization, and maintenance of cooking skills. *Journal of Behavioral Education, 4*, 283–311.

Troia, G. A., & Graham, S. (2002). The effectiveness of a highly explicit, teacher-directed strategy instruction routine: Changing the writing performance of students with learning disabilities. *Journal of Learning Disabilities, 35*, 290–305.

Tymchuk, A. J. (1985). *Effective decision making for the developmentally disabled.* Portland, OR: EDNICK Communications, Inc.

Tymchuk, A. J., Andron, L., & Rahbar, B. (1988). Effective decision-making problem-solving training with mothers who have mental retardation. *American Journal on Mental Retardation, 92*, 510–516.

Tymchuk, A. J., Yokota, A., & Rahbar, B. (1990). Decision-making abilities of mothers with mental retardation. *Research in Developmental Disabilities, 11*, 97–109.

Vac, N. A., Vallecorsa, A. L., Parker, A., Bonner, S., Lester, C., Richardson, S., et al. (1985). Parents' and educators' participation in IEP conferences. *Education and Treatment of Children, 8*, 153–162.

Valenzuela, R. L., & Martin, J. E. (2005). The self-directed IEP: Bridging values of diverse cultures and secondary education. *Career Development for Exceptional Individuals, 28*, 4–14.

Van Dycke, J. L. (2005). *Determining the impact of the Self-Directed IEP instruction on secondary IEP documents.* Unpublished doctoral dissertation, University of Oklahoma, Norman.

Van Dycke, J. L., Lovett, D. L., Greene, B. A., & Martin, J. E. (2006). *Opening a window into secondary teacher-directed IEP transition meetings: Whose voices are we hearing?* Manuscript submitted for publication.

Vygotsky, L. S. (1962). *Thought and language.* Cambridge, MA: MIT Press.

Wacker, D. P., Berg, W. K., McMahon, C., Templeman, M., McKinney, J., Swarts, V., et al. (1988). An evaluation of labeling-then-doing with moderately handicapped persons: Acquisition and generalization with complex tasks. *Journal of Applied Behavior Analysis, 21*, 369–380.

Wacker, D., Berg, W., Wiggins, B., Muldoon, M., & Cavanaugh, J. (1985). Evaluation of reinforcer preference for profoundly handicapped students. *Journal of Applied Behavior Analysis, 18*, 173–178.

Wacker, D. P., Carroll, J. L., & Moe, G. L. (1980). Acquisition, generalization, and maintenance of an assembly task by mentally retarded children. *American Journal of Mental Deficiency, 85*, 286–290.

Wacker, D. P., & Greenebaum, F. T. (1984). Efficacy of a verbal training sequence on the sorting performance of moderately and severely mentally retarded adolescents. *American Journal of Mental Deficiency, 88,* 653–660.

Wacker, D. P., Wiggins, B., Fowler, M., & Berg, W. K. (1988). Training students with profound or multiple handicaps to make requests via microswitches. *Journal of Applied Behavior Analysis, 21,* 331–343.

Wagner, W., Newman, L., Cameto, R., & Levine, P. (2005). Changes over time in the early postschool outcomes of youth with disabilities. *A report of findings from the National Longitudinal Transition Study (NLTS) and National Longitudinal Transition Study-2 (NLTS2).* Menlo Park, CA: SRI International. Retrieved January 25, 2006 from *www.nlts2.org/*

Ward, M. J. (2005). An historical perspective on self-determination in special education: Accomplishments and challenges. *Research and Practice for Persons with Severe Disabilities, 30,* 108–112.

Warner, D. A., & DeJung, J. E. (1971). Effects of goal setting upon learning in educable retardates. *American Journal of Mental Deficiency, 75,* 681–684.

Watanabe, M., & Sturmey, P. (2003). The effect of choice-making opportunities during activity schedules on task engagement of adults with autism. *Journal of Autism and Developmental Disorders, 33,* 535–538.

Wehmeyer, M. L. (1992a). Self-determination: Critical skills for outcome-oriented transition services. *Journal for Vocational Special Needs Education, 39,* 153–163.

Wehmeyer, M. L. (1992b). Self-determination and the education of students with mental retardation. *Education and Training in Mental Retardation, 27,* 302–314.

Wehmeyer, M. L. (1996). A self-report measure of self-determination for adolescents with cognitive disabilities. *Education and Training in Mental Retardation and Developmental Disabilities, 31,* 282–293.

Wehmeyer, M. L. (2001). Self-determination and mental retardation. In L. M. Glidden (Ed.), *International review of research in mental retardation* (Vol. 24, pp. 1–48). San Diego, CA: Academic Press.

Wehmeyer, M. L. (2002). The confluence of person-centered planning and self-determination. In S. Holburn & P. M. Vietze (Eds.), *Person-centered planning* (pp. 51–72). Baltimore: Brookes.

Wehmeyer, M. L. (2005). Self-determination and individuals with severe disabilities: Re-examining meanings and misinterpretations. *Research and Practice for Persons with Severe Disabilities, 30,* 112–120.

Wehmeyer, M. L. (2006). Self-determination and individuals with severe disabilities: Reexamining meanings and misinterpretations. *Research and Practice in Severe Disabilities, 30,* 113–120.

Wehmeyer, M. L., Abery, B., Mithaug, D. E., & Stancliffe, R. J. (2003). *Theory in self-determination: Foundations for educational practice.* Springfield, IL: Thomas.

Wehmeyer, M. L., Agran, M., & Hughes, C. (1998). *Teaching self-determination to students with disabilities: Basic skills for successful transition.* Baltimore: Brookes.

Wehmeyer, M. L., Agran, M., & Hughes, C. (2000). A national survey of teachers' promotion of self-determination and student-directed learning. *Journal of Special Education, 34,* 58–68.

Wehmeyer, M. L., Agran, M., Palmer, S. B., & Mithaug, D. (1999). *A teacher's guide to implementing the self-determined learning model of instruction: Adolescent version.* Lawrence, KS: Self-Determination Projects, Beach Center on Families and Disability, Schiefelbusch Institute for Life Span Studies, University of Kansas.

Wehmeyer, M. L., & Berkobien, R. (1996). The legacy of self-advocacy: People with cognitive disabilities as leaders in their community. In G. Dybwad & H. Bersani (Eds.), *New voices: Self-advocacy by people with disabilities* (pp. 246–257). Cambridge, MA: Brookline.

Wehmeyer, M. L., Field, S., Doren, B., Jones, B., & Mason, C. (2004). Self-determination and student involvement in standards-based reform. *Exceptional Children, 70*, 413–425.

Wehmeyer, M. L., Hughes, C., Agran, M., Garner, N., & Yeager, D. (2003). Student-directed learning strategies to promote the progress of students with intellectual disability in inclusive classrooms. *International Journal of Inclusive Education, 7*, 415–428.

Wehmeyer, M. L., & Kelchner, K. (1994). Interpersonal cognitive problem-solving skills of individuals with mental retardation. *Education and Training in Mental Retardation and Developmental Disabilities, 29*, 265–278.

Wehmeyer, M. L., Kelchner, K., & Richards, S. (1995). Individual and environmental factors related to the self-determination of adults with mental retardation. *Journal of Vocational Rehabilitation, 5*, 291–305.

Wehmeyer, M. L., Kelchner, K., & Richards. S. (1996). Essential characteristics of self-determined behaviors of adults with mental retardation and developmental disabilities. *American Journal of Mental Retardation, 100*, 632–642.

Wehmeyer, M. L., & Lawrence, M. (1995). Whose future is it anyway?: Promoting student involvement in transition planning. *Career Development for Exceptional Individuals, 18*, 69–83.

Wehmeyer, M. L., & Lawrence, M. (in press). A national replication of a student-directed transition-planning process: Impact on student knowledge of and perceptions about transition planning. *Education and Treatment of Children.*

Wehmeyer, M. L., Lawrence, M., Kelchner, K., Palmer, S., Garner, N., & Soukup, J. (2004). *Whose future is it anyway: A student-directed transition-planning process* (2nd ed.). Lawrence, KS: Beach Center on Disability.

Wehmeyer, M. L., & Metzler, C. (1995). How self-determined are people with mental retardation? The National Consumer Survey. *Mental Retardation, 33*, 111–119.

Wehmeyer, M. L., & Palmer, S. (2003). Adult outcomes for students with cogntive disabilities three years after high school: The impact of self-determination. *Education and Training in Developmental Disabilities, 38*(2), 131–144.

Wehmeyer, M. L., Palmer, S. B., Agran, M., Mithaug, D. E., & Martin, J. E. (2000). Promoting causal agency: The self-determined learning model of instruction. *Exceptional Children, 66*, 439–453.

Wehmeyer, M. L., Palmer, S., Smith, S., Parent, W., Davies, D. K., & Stock, S. (2006). Technology use by people with intellectual and developmental disabilities to support employment activities: A single-subject design meta analysis. *Journal of Vocational Rehabilitation, 24*, 81–86.

Wehmeyer, M. L., Sands, D. J., Doll, B., & Palmer, S. (1997). The development of self-determination and implications for educational interventions with students with disabilities. *International Journal of Disability, Development and Education, 44*, 305–328.

Wehmeyer, M. L., & Schwartz, M. (1997). Self-determination and positive adult outcomes: A follow-up study of youth with mental retardation or learning disabilities. *Exceptional Children, 63*(2), 245–255.

Wehmeyer, M. L., & Schwartz, M. (1998). The relationship between self-determination and quality of life for adults with mental retardation. *Education and Training in Mental Retardation and Developmental Disabilities, 33*(1), 3–12.

Wehmeyer, M. L., Smith, S. J., & Davies, D. K. (2005). Technology use and students with intellectual disability: Universal design for all students. In D. Edyburn, K. Higgins, & R. Boone (Eds.), *Handbook of special education technology research and practice* (pp. 309–323). Whitefish Bay, WI: Knowledge by Design.

Wehmeyer, M. L., Smith, S. J., Palmer, S. B., Davies, D. K., & Stock, S. (2004). Technology use and people with mental retardation. In L. M. Glidden (Ed.), *International review of research in mental retardation* (Vol. 29, pp. 293–337). San Diego: Academic Press.

Wehmeyer, M. L., Yeager, D., Wade, N., Agran, M., & Hughes, C. (2003). The effects of self-regulation strategies on goal attainment for students with developmental disabilities in general education classrooms. *Journal of Developmental and Physical Disabilities, 15,* 79–91.

West, L. L., Corbey, S., Boyer-Stephens, A., Jones, B., Miller, R. J., & Sarkees-Wircenski, M. (1992). *Integrating transition planning into the IEP process.* Reston, VA: Council for Exceptional Children.

Whitman, T. L. (1990). Self-regulation and mental retardation. *American Journal of Mental Retardation, 94,* 347–362.

Whitman, T. L., & Johnston, M. B. (1983). Teaching addition and subtraction with regrouping to educable mentally retarded children: A group self-instructional training program. *Behavior Therapy, 14,* 127–143.

Williams, J. M., & O'Leary, E. (2001). What we've learned and where we go from here. *Career Development for Exceptional Individuals, 24*(1), 51–71.

Winking, D., O'Reilly, B., & Moon, M. (1993). Preference: The missing link in the job match process for individuals without functional communication skills. *Journal of Vocational Rehabilitation, 3,* 27–42.

Wolpe, J. (1969). *The practice of behavior therapy.* Oxford, UK: Pergamon Press.

Wolpe, J., & Lazarus, A.A. (1966). *Behavior therapy techniques: A guide to the treatment of neuroses.* Oxford, UK: Pergamon Press.

Wood, W. M., Fowler, C. H., Uphold, N., & Test, D. W. (2005). A review of self-determination interventions with individuals with severe disabilities. *Research and Practice for Persons with Severe Disabilities, 30,* 121–146.

Woods, L. L., & Martin, J. E. (2004). Improving supervisor evaluations through the use of self-determination contracts. *Career Development for Exceptional Individuals, 27,* 207–220.

Woodward, J., Carnine, D., & Bersten, R. (1988). Teaching problem solving through computer simulations. *American Educational Research Journal, 25,* 72–86.

Wu, P., Martin, J. E., & Isabell, S. (2006). *Increasing participation of students who are blind or visually impaired in their IEP meetings.* Manuscript submitted for publication.

Wuerch, B. B., & Voeltz, L. M. (1982). *Longitudinal leisure skills for severely handicapped learners: The Ho 'onanea curriculum component.* Baltimore: Brookes.

Zaragoza, N., Vaughn, S., & McIntosh, R. (1991). Social skills interventions and children with behavior problems: A review. *Behavioral Disorders, 16,* 260–275.

Zhang, D. (2001). The effect of 'Next S.T.E.P.' instruction on the self-determination skills of high school students with learning disabilities. *Career Development for Exceptional Individuals, 24,* 121–132.

Zhang, D. (2005). Parent practices in facilitating self-determination skills: The influence of culture, socioeconomic status, and children's special education status. *Research and Practice for Persons with Severe Disabilities, 30,* 154–162.

Zhang, D., Wehmeyer, M. L., & Chen, L.J. (2005). Parent and teacher engagement in fostering the self-determination of students with disabilities: A comparison between the U.S. and the Republic of China. *Remedial and Special Education, 26,* 55–64.

Zimmerman, B., Bandura, A., & Martinez-Pons, M. (1992). Self-motivation for academic attainment: The role of self-efficacy beliefs and personal goal setting. *American Educational Research Journal, 29,* 663–676.

Zimmerman, B. J., Bonner, S., & Kovach, R. (1996). *Developing self-regulated learners: Beyond achievement to self-efficacy.* Washington, DC: American Psychological Association.

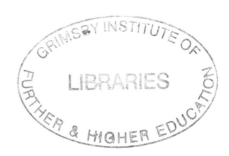

Index

"f" following a page number indicates a figure; "t" following a page number indicates a table.